The Healthcare Practitioners Guide to Conflict Engagement and Dispute Resolution

Michael Schneider MD, FACS, MS-ADR

Copyright © 2018 Medport Publishing

ISBN-10: 0692136053
ISBN-13: 978-0692136058

This textbook covers critical information applicable to daily disagreements between staff,

partnership disputes, contract negotiations, and tort claims management for medical practitioners.

The information will improve the quality of the medical practice, patient safety and the practitioner's sense of professional fulfilment in a healthcare system dynamically changing and embroiled in complex and protracted conflict.

Dedication –

To Michelle,

who taught me to quiet the demons, cool my jets, find peace, and enjoy every moment.

The Healthcare Practitioners Guide to
Conflict Engagement and Dispute Resolution

Michael Schneider MD FACS MS-ADR
7/2018
First Edition

ISBN-13: 978-0692136058
ISBN-10: 0692136053

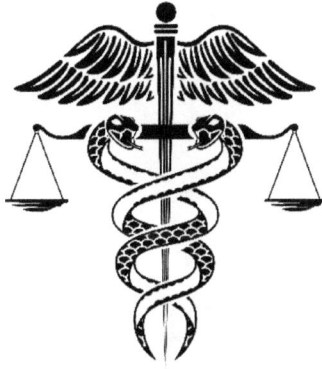

Table of Contents

PREFACE

This book introduces healthcare practitioners to the field of conflict engagement and dispute resolution. This text will improve your professional relationships. Research demonstrates these skills benefit the practitioner's own sense of success and wellbeing while dramatically reducing errors in patient care. The academic discipline of Alternative Dispute Resolution, or ADR, offered as graduate level training through colleges and law centers, provides both skills development and insight into effective dispute management systems. Providers are far better off when they successfully manage contentious professional conversations with resolution and collaboration. By employing non-adverse techniques and changing the narrative, the provider learns to meet their own needs and interests while facilitating the interests of one's opponents.

This information is part of the educational curriculum and expectations of postgraduate medical training and licensure. Every person in healthcare should dedicate time and effort to master these communication skills. In this manual, the definition of healthcare providers includes all technicians, therapists, nursing, mid-levels and doctors who together, comprise the integrated team members determining the quality and safety of a patient's experience. The life and health of the individual and the entire organization can only succeed when professional relationships are expressive and healthy discourse resolves conflict. As social creatures, we must provide attention, respect, agency and have insight into our opponent's positions and recognize their contribution to the medical community. Only recently are some healthcare institutions advocating, through administrative imperative, an integrated conflict management system (ICMS) which is a graduated approach for addressing disputes. At its lowest level, only the arguing parties are involved. Individuals are encouraged to try and speak to the person they perceive offended them. Because of this, some organizations implementing an ICMS system offer communication skills work-shops, teaching employees critical techniques to give and receive effective feedback and constructive criticism. Within ICMS, if one to one dialogue fails, then facilitators and mediators get involved. Ultimately, failed resolution usually triggers arbitrated case management, attempting to expedite conflict resolution and diminish the expensive adversarial and public embarrassment of a litigated court case. The ICMS approach requires education and training, identifying and resolving disagreements at the least adversarial and most constructive level possible.

In healthcare, major universities are beginning to integrate medically specific conflict resolution skills development and providing advanced training to enhance educational opportunities for those interested in this field, including careers in healthcare mediation and arbitration. The deceptively simple goal is to improve safe and superior medical care, minimizing adverse events and improving professional collegiality. The highest levels of the discipline are routinely used when managing potential or real litigation. Within the profession of alternative dispute resolution (ADR), the spectrum of services offered from a conflict management specialist extend from communication skills training that empowers the individual, through sophisticated arbitration in lieu of court litigated cases. Today, the healthcare professional must utilize their working knowledge of fundamental concepts in dispute resolution to hopefully prevent adverse and contentious positions. When conflicts arise, the provider must understand the nuances, benefits and pitfalls of the mediation and arbitration process.

This textbook is appropriate for providers, administrators and legal advocates. The educational goals and reasons to complete this study include:

1. A fundamental understanding of the discipline of conflict management and dispute resolution and its practical influence on the personal and professional lives of healthcare providers.

2. An academic exposure and practicum example of conflict scenarios assessed through alternative discourse. Through study, the individual develops skills to preemptively manage routine conflicts and this text provides a compelling resource for systems and methods applied to resolve common disputes in the healthcare profession.

Acknowledgment

The author must recognize the excellent work and assistance of members of medical staff services and risk management departments at Creighton University Healthcare Center in Omaha Nebraska. This physician author is grateful for their insight and assistance in my own master's program education and I pay them the highest respect for their dedication to healthcare provider well-being, and as excellent patient advocates executing the highest quality of healthcare delivery. In my experience as a physician, reiterated at this institution, the offices of risk management are at the ground level to investigate and implement a platform for conflict management, educating providers to recognize and develop skills in this discipline.

Chapter One

Conflict in the life of the Healthcare Provider

Medical education and professional practice experience hardens our emotional and psychological defenses. The pace is intense and chaotic. Providers are forced to master an overwhelming body of knowledge and chastised for the slightest error or omission. Repeated daily, the practitioner's success demands complex and logical analysis while disregarding the personal emotional impact of stress, disappointment, morbidity and mortality. The healthcare professional must suppress their emotional inclination, their displays of sorrow, empathy and compassion in order to survive. Feelings don't reveal a diagnosis, order a test, or interpret a lab result. Feelings have no weight on rounds and there are no E & M code or CPT codes to quantify our expressions of benevolence. The provider creates barriers to insulate against guilt or shame if treatment does not produce the desired result. Along the way, we disengage from non-clinical language and discourse and our communication skills falter. We interpret argument and negotiations as a linear endeavor relying on scientific and didactic methodology to arrive at our preconceived version of truth. We attempt to persuade or browbeat our conclusions into indisputable facts so that we may move on to the next emergency. Conflict management skills training is irrelevant to our professional practice yet here we are, steeped in disputes between providers, administrators, and patients who are now plaintiff's. How we arrived is illogical and disregards our effort and dedication to our calling, our passion, and our professionalism. The mental energy is exhausting as we fixate on the conflict, convinced of our debate superiority and confident we will dominate any conversation because we are a respected healthcare professional.

Why bother reading on then? This textbook will not reset the reader's moral compass or alter behavior by generating commanding authoritative principals, such as: be kinder, walk softer, and be more understanding. Instead, consider conflict management education as an academic case management exercise, where we identify the pathology causing conflict; dissect into its pathophysiology through discourse between key stake-holder individuals; then define a treatment plan, where our role as providers integrates our knowledge and effort to stop the anger and divisive behavior which hemorrhages our civility. Therefore, as a professional in the healthcare field, perhaps the incentive to study this information and incorporate these new skills, recognizes that refinement of our persona demands personal responsibility to manage conflict similar to any disease we encounter. Conflict engagement and dispute resolution requires recognition, acknowledgment, and transference of adversarial persuasion expressed through empathy. Discovering the tools and applications successful for these skills requires study and practice. One of the most important tools a skilled conflict manager develops, as exemplified throughout this text, is reframing techniques.

A frame is simply the perception of events. Since conflict stimulates a visceral defensive recoil in most people, the skill to reframe perceptions is critical. Reframing is altering filters in parties, deliberately changing views and interpretation of events. Reframing energy expressed by adversaries provides hope while mitigating the stress of disputes, stimulating resourcefulness when faced with a significant challenge. As skilled provider-managers, we assume control of the intervention, modify the treatment plan as needed and resolve the conflict, returning parties to a stable steady-state. In post procedure rounds, we might implement some preventative care through communication management to avoid the recidivism of traumatic conflict. Our payment for services will be a productive and efficient interpersonal professional work environment where our needs, like respect, identification of our expertise and authority in our field, as well as our autonomy, all coincide. Success is dispute management engenders gratitude from one's colleagues, recognizing that effective resolution directly improves the actual patient care experience and the quality of the organizational care delivery at the healthcare institution.

The many theories in alternative dispute resolution are not debated or vetted in this book. Excellent resources are cataloged in the bibliography for the student anxious to expand their understanding of the practical application of behavior psychology during conflict situations, and how to manage the consequences of disagreement. Instead, this thesis focuses on practical management techniques by presenting common scenarios that are typical of mis-communication and positional demands between providers. We stop and reframe the conflict scenario utilizing an academic exercise for both on-the-fly and deeper analysis, showing the provider techniques and strategies to manage these conflicts. It is important to have a reflective acknowledgment that although we may not believe our personalities and communication skills stimulate conflict, that is rarely the case. In a hierarchical system in which years of education and responsibility separate different healthcare providers, acknowledging this power differential is critical. Developing skills in communication management through inquisitive investigation will reveal interests that are often quite similar, allowing healthcare providers to move forward in a new storyline of professional integrity and respect. This is proven to result in safer medical care delivery.

Alternative dispute resolution studies provide a rich background and understanding for the psychology behind conflict, the essence of conflict escalation, including common attribution errors like prejudice and blaming. ADR studies both the degree of resolution and methods designed toward de-escalating conflict through communication and trust building. By appreciating the discourse of ADR theories, we begin to understand that language and cultural norms shape both individual and group behavior bringing them into conflict with alternative cultures. In addition, dynamics that significantly influence understanding and reaction to a conflict occur because of gender, socioeconomic status, and race. In healthcare, we see all these factors combined with an effective hierarchical and authoritative sub cultural that dominates and frames the spectrum of conflicts, from simple miscommunication to the extremes of litigated disputes. Most of us approach conflict as a win - lose proposition instead of an integrative problem-solving collaboration, allowing us to work in concert with our opponent, improving both of our situations through a win-win proposition.

There is a continuum of dispute resolution models to study and implement. The spectrum includes effective negotiation between parties, parties use of a non-neutral assistant in some capacity (facilitators), various types of mediation where the third-party is neutral and impartial or may provide facilitative insight but defer solutions to the opponent parties. Lastly, disputes may rely upon a more formal process of adjudication, using private adjudication through a variety of contract arbitrations or deferring to the public court system. In addition, ADR techniques in community government often regulate by consensus or majority vote, establishing rules and laws requiring individual compliance.

The essence of negotiation when a dispute arises, sees individuals who either claim value, wishing only to receive the largest part of the fixed reward, and those who see conflict as a method to increase a shared value with creation of greater opportunities that allow all parties to benefit from the relationship. Perceived authority or power and political differentials, ethics, morals and past and future relationship play significant parts in how we approach negotiation. During negotiation, we might implore a third party to assist in the process, however when a third-party is coaching and advocating for one party's reward at the expense of another, they are facilitating one sides' claims and not mediating a dispute. Regardless, active communication requires dialogue. An effective dialogue can only begin by quieting prejudice and bias between parties. Effective dialogue requires active listening, empathy, and the ability to discount one's own belief system based upon normative cultural values. The individual must grant authority and permission for an alternative viewpoint to interpret the same facts and situation that created the dispute.

Dialogue in essence is learning and requires receptive interpretation of disputed issues by alternative sources, suspending our potentially limited positional opinions while not abandoning our own committed interests. In effect, dialogue requires all parties to express self-interests but accept an alternative conclusion once credence and authority are granted to another's views. Parties in conflict exposed to well-constructed dialogue framework often embrace humanism for the greater good. Be wary though, as any technique that assumes that self-interest will not trump communal resolution must be approached fastidiously. In societies that celebrate personal power, material possessions, and authoritative rule, pure altruism is a precious rare gem. In reality, most people in power generally relish and protect the perception of power. In any culture rewarding individualism there exists a symbiotic cohabitation with social and cultural order by persons who search for opportunity for individual gain and greater power. Those entrenched perspectives will challenge the value of discourse and dialogue.

The process of dispute mediation might be evaluative where the opinion of a mediator is requested by both parties, or facilitative, in which the mediator utilizes strategies and techniques for conflict analysis without rendering their opinion. Regardless of orientation, mediators do not provide solutions. These are generated by the conflicting parties. Also, true mediation requires the third-party neutral to be disengaged and not benefit from or have a specific interest in the outcome of the mediated process. In healthcare, a doctor, nurse, or administrator who assumes the mediator position does have a tangential interest in a civil outcome – peace and improved patient care. Thus in medicine, wearing the hat of the mediator during a dispute is acceptable as long as one party's position is not advocated by the mediator. The mediator is within their authority when reminding parties that the mission of the institution, to provide quality healthcare, superseded the individual interests of either opponent.

There is a spectrum of mediation styles including positional, facilitative, narrative and transformative approaches and techniques. Many of the differences relate to the depth of understanding of needs and interests by the parties and how the opponents communicate their desires. Often the back story and past experiences between the disputing parties are deep and convoluted and approaches such as the transformative mediation style spends an enormous amount of time ferreting out the inner emotions and perceptions of adversaries, seeking to change the individual's fundamental view of the conflict and alter the very nature of the relationship, establishing default collaboration when these parties meet in future conflict. In medicine, given the time constraints and the required quick evaluate and expedited dispositional demands (each party expressing their view while claiming their needs), several methods are reviewed in this textbook, enabling the provider with the quick and practical skills of conflict identification, analysis and management. This improves and empowers communication, strengthens negotiation, and teaches methods to de-escalate arguments. These goals support a collaborative attempt to establish and maintain an excellent working environment, free of oppression, retaliation, and fear while concentrating on the complex task of efficient, rewarding and quality healthcare delivery.

Interest-based negotiation evokes a wide range of human response. The intent is to engage in problem solving that elevates and responds to the breadth of those interests, and in the process to invent added options for settlement. By attending to interests, parties can resolve a broader spectrum of issues, expand choices and settle their dispute through a more fulfilling experience for mutual benefit. Interest-based negotiation defines an approach to the process of expanding and exchanging both tangibles and intangibles. Rather than regarding each other as contestants, interest-based negotiators associate as collaborators, seeking overlapping objectives. Recognizing their interdependence, they discover that they both win by advocating for their opponents' wellbeing and satisfactory outcome. Out of the process of building trust and open communication, they derive genuine confidence that extends well beyond any single transaction.

Interest-based negotiation is particularly compelling when parties are engaged in tasks that elicit their underlying objectives, or their sense of purpose, as is typical in the work of healthcare. It is especially pragmatic when there are limited resources to divide, frequently encountered in the medical environment. Creative collaborative investigation often expands those limited assets utility and efficiently shares those assets to meet the needs of all parties. Despite this model's inherent utility for health care, there are those who shun it, preferring a win-lose, competitive approach instead.

The earlier we incorporate constructive resolution, the less likely these disagreements will escalate. Nevertheless, when heated disputes do arise, an easily accessible and pragmatic mediation procedure is a useful and efficient way to bring parties to the negotiation table. In healthcare, conflicts and their resolution are a vital source of invaluable information about issues that might improve the quality of patient care or of staff members' work lives. When the dispute or problem involves an error that reduces patient safety, one point of the settlement is typically system changes that eliminate the possibility that the same error will be committed by someone else. The essence of the root cause analysis investigation arises from an acknowledged conflict in which the system itself may be at fault.

When former disputants resume a close working relationship or when someone must return to the circumstances that generated the dispute in the first place, the lessons learned must be incorporated into a reformed practice style and system design. When a practitioner returns to routine patient care following a malpractice case with one patient, when nurses resume collaborative work following a dispute with the medical staff, or when administrators reestablish business ties following a disputed issue with a vendor, what follows that resolution must be different matured behavior between all vested parties. It is essential to ask: How can we prevent the same dispute or problem occurring again? This question becomes a routine aspect of the settlement process, so that systemic learning amplifies the value of the settlement. In other words, the evaluation and solution are shared throughout the system so all stakeholders in the larger complex understand the issues and avoid conflict or mistakes because of new awareness. In this way conflict management can be helpful well beyond the culmination of a single dispute.

The willingness to change perspective will only arise when healthcare providers actively participate in reflective practice. The reflective introspective inquiry is the ability to contemplate on one's actions and behavior as a process of continuous learning, acknowledging our own values, prejudices, and perceptions which dictate our daily conduct, and define our character. Our goals toward self-actualization improves our sense of self-worth, our community mind and our interpersonal skills when collaborating on patient care. As expected from studies on human nature, when we achieve success through hard work, we expect autonomy, respect and authority. Without contempt or condescension, we are entitled to social gratitude and recognition, taking pride in our own efforts, commitment and accomplishment. When we demand respect and authority however, we are perceived as positional, defensive, arrogant and authoritative. We often ignore the knowledge and experience of our personal and professional circle. Practically speaking, trying to reject the team concept of healthcare integration and preserve hierarchical authority based upon institutional achievement, is a threat to quality patient management. These behaviors are nearly universally rejected and constitute the foundation of dispute instigation in Medicine. Our willingness to be reflective in our own practice of communication and interaction with our colleagues at all levels of training is critical for our personal success, free from cognitive turmoil and dissonance, and in that success our professionalism will drive us to provide the highest quality of attentive patient care.

Academic analysis shows us that common dispositional demands from people in a traditional hierarchical system like healthcare results from their defensiveness and fear of having made a mistake, guilt and or fear of shame, as well as attribution errors (blaming others or the situation) from myopic approaches to problems. Practitioners have become so used to the conflict narrative in medicine that aggressive positional behavior and demands, occurring all around us, no longer register in our mind as emotionally driven by adverse parties. The provider becomes numb and distant to the emotional impact conflict has on ourselves and our closest relationships, both professionally and personally, from our adaptation to the intense clinical work space. However, not everyone in this work place is equally insulated, so the emotional and visceral consequences of heated discussions, yelling, and angry debate influences and stresses many in the field. Likely, it is also subliminally affecting us and fueling our malaise, burnout and antipathy toward the profession of medicine. The apathy we feel over a day in clinic or responsive anger to the 11pm call to clarify an order is founded in the impact of these daily angry disputes. The conflict narrative causes replay event psychological fixation with our ever-improving clever positional responses, all disrupting peace of mind and a restful night's sleep. At times this fixation is pathological, and we cannot quiet our mind and refocus our attention. We accept the dysthymic and depressive influence this has on our mood and behavior as we bury the distaste deep in our subconscious. These are fundamental conditions for post-traumatic stress disorder.

The effort of this text is therefore to educate and arm the practitioner with knowledge-based skills in interest-based collaboration. As mediators will represent, all parties do benefit when creative solutions are developed and ratified by opponents and the dispute situation is not attributed to character flaws by either conflicted party. Also, each argument is adequately unique and should not be forced to resort to limited strict rules of case law when developing solutions. When the provider finds himself in conflict, attempt to de-escalate and resolve issues using the following strategies: enhanced communication, trust building and integrative problem solving. Improved communication requires a party to suspend judgement and engage in active listening. Doug Stone notes that miscommunication and mis judgements typically see a party try and justify their position over and over, arguing because the other side is wrong in a "them vs us" mentality. Arguing without truly understanding the nature of a dispute is circular and unlikely to resolve any issues. So, listen attentively to your opponent and discover how they came to their conclusions. Request the same courtesy from them.

Acknowledging the needs and interests of patients affected by adverse outcomes with empathy and apology is very effective. Helpful phrases include: *"I want to say how sorry I am for what happened, and I hear you say...;"* *"...you are concerned about the long-term consequences for your family member (patient);"* *"...you worry about who will pay for the extra care"; "...you feel like someone should be held accountable for what happened"; "you want information about how this could have happened."* During your conversation respond to emotional outbursts with: *" I can see that you are upset/unhappy/worried/angry..."; "I imagine you may feel like...".* Recognize the difference between an empathetic or partial apology, one that apologizes for the situation and impact on the patient without claiming responsibility, vs an apology of responsibility, such as *"I'm sorry we did this to you..."* Although the full apology is protected from disclosure in many states, always review this issue with risk management and hospital counsel before offering this concession. Also recognize that when adverse outcomes occur, there are ethical and legal doctrine that require some type of disclosure. The reader may reference the standards, statutes and ethics requiring disclosure found in the Joint Commission standards and elements of performance, the AMA code of medical ethics, the American College of Physicians ethics manual and the ACOG committee opinion. Disclosure and the role of the dispute resolution specialist are discussed extensively throughout this textbook.

By incorporating the objectives in this textbook, and hopefully your new learner perspective, think of skill development in interest-based communication from the mediator lens as catharsis in professional discourse, maintaining the control and direction of resolution.

Really, is this any different than our need to influence and exercise control over pathology that ravages the body or mind? Providers, whether dentists, chiropractors, nurses, mid-levels, surgeons or medical providers, implicitly believe they have patient care and safety as their primary directive. This is the foundational statement defining our identity. To serve and heal, an ethic allowing our survival through brutal years of education and ongoing success in a high conflict, intense and unforgiving environment.

Nevertheless, we name and blame mistakes on "others" caused by simple miscommunication or dismiss and devalue positions that are not in line with our own thinking. The individuals on the other side can quickly transition from colleague and compatriot to opponent and enemy even when long standing work relationships were healthy. In conflict, we rarely see and certainly won't admit that our assumption of the other party's intentions were anything but malignant and self-serving. We attribute our actions as righteous and benevolent and the opponents as divisive and uneducated. We quickly escalate conflict from our doing well and winning the argument, to winning and hurting the other person before we can claim victory. People who are angry and in dispute limit and alter their communication pattern and this creates undo risk to patient care and quality initiatives. Think of simple examples of failed communication and consequences: a nurse vs. nurse issue when passing on a patient during shift change; a PA to physician issue about an unexpected vital sign that the PA misinterprets; between doctors when one demands a patient a treatment but the other demands to follow a different treatment regimen.

Just because we can scream that our position is always right 'based on our experience' or 'the literature says,' healthcare is rarely immutable. Very few academic positions are authoritative and define absolute standard of care for every pathology and issue. In fact, most national colleges and organizations are very specific to say their recommendations are only guidelines. In legal cases, the standard of care is defined as what is reasonable for someone with similar training and experience to do under the same circumstances as the provider. As professionals we are self-confident that in our practices we deliver treatment superior to any "standard of care", thus when a colleague has an alternative treatment course, we angerly defend our position. But consider, aren't both parties trying to affect a similar outcome? When do extreme positions inspire communication with other healthcare professionals also claiming their approach is absolutely definitive? The result of course, is narrow-minded execution of a care pathway that fails to integrate experience and alternative important perspectives.

As the care recipients, patients and families become confused and concerned. These dependent beneficiaries sense dispersions between providers and their trust, which is tenuous at best, results in panic and misperception. They then exhibit their own extreme defensive and demanding claims. And when the doctors/PA/NP leaves the room, who do they assault with their fears and worry - the nurses! The impact of unresolved and hostile positioning by professionals does directly influence the quality of care for the patient, even if it by subsequent psychological impact of the hostile exchange, and not resultant from actual mistakes in case management. Through generalization, families and patients blame the facility and all associated providers, claiming loudly they are collectively inferior. In a day where social media impacts our practice, we really cannot afford these pervasive and destructive conflicts threatening the unity concept of quality healthcare management.

The employees in conflict (or the employee who creates a "toxic environment" in the workplace) creates a negative atmosphere for their coworkers that hurts morale and subverts the quality patient experience. High turnover rates are costly and when people quit or are fired because of behavioral problems, the cost to the organization is profound. Joint Commission on Accreditation of Healthcare Organizations (JCAHO) is mandating that hospitals manage conflict in a way that healthcare safety and quality are protected while diminishing work place violence. Human resource departments are adopting a zero-tolerance policy to interpersonal conflicts due to the rise of "hostile work environment" lawsuits.

The underlying theme in this textbook are founded in generativity theory, to create a legacy enabling providers to avoid the mistakes the author witnessed or made over a thirty-year neurosurgery career. Please begin by learning the art of active listening. Empathetic attention during conversation reveals your opponent's perspective and dismisses your urge to interrupt, qualify, and correct their understanding of events or issues. In time you will develop a deeper appreciation of inclusion, diversity of views, perspective and become tolerant of opinions that may differ, recognizing that in the end, we all have common needs, interests and goals. Combining the tools of leadership, adherence to policy, and working from an interest-based perspective, healthcare providers learn how to work through the inevitable issues that occur while caring for patients. By proactively addressing problematic situations you will receive a profoundly valuable personal payoff – reduced stress and wasted time, efficient accurate patient care, and comfortable, rewarding professional satisfaction.

The conflicts scenarios in the final appendix of this text may reveal some personal identification and stimulate introspective practice analysis. These dispute challenges are academic exercises preparing the practitioner to engage future arguments with a reflective and methodical approach. Skill development ensures that future challenges or questions about your professional decisions by patients, colleagues or administrative bodies, are effectively managed utilizing dispute resolution techniques. This ability will effectively disarm your opponent's tirade and deflate a demanding and confrontational high conflict personality terrorizing the clinic or operating room.

To be effective, people must suppress their own difficult personality traits and develop alternative communication strategies. To reiterate the content of this treatise, spend a few moments practicing these communication techniques. Consider hostile and dysfunctional argumentative attacks as a communicable disease; first recognized, then analyzed, and finally eradicated to avoid its toxic spread to everyone else in your environment. Treat the hosts by managing the interests and expression of need by your adversaries. Try facilitating small and large group conflict resolution. Explore through dynamic discourse, the articulation of individual and then group overlapping collaborative interests, moving the conversation to a unique narrative. Cure the pathology that generated the dispute with options that meet expectations and resolve interests, while inoculating to suppress malignant positional demands. As we know, success in disease recognition, management and remedy is uniquely fulfilling as a healthcare practitioner.

Chapter2

Interpersonal friction, conflict and fulfilling our needs and interests

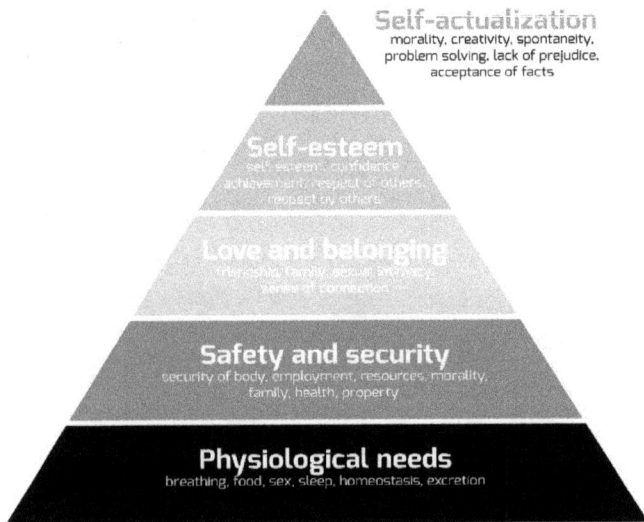

Who created this dispute?

Human beings, particularly motivated individuals pursuing careers in healthcare, possess an innate desire to achieve their highest potential. We must attend to our basic needs and defend our respective wellbeing, while professional challenges and interpersonal conflicts inevitably interrupt this pursuit.

Psychologist Abraham Maslow studied and described the foundations of human needs using a pyramidal formulation which requires both achievement and stability of subordinate needs before a person could progress toward the apex of self-actualization. Conflict in our lives distracts from our journey and entraps our attention and emotion, stifling progress and threatening contentment. Maslow demonstrated that needs can be both tangible and psychological, and that progressive accomplishment of goals and desires results in individual happiness and fulfillment.

At the pyramid base are requirements for the organisms survival, such as physical needs of food and shelter. With these secure, we pursue security interests such as protection from violence, and a safe and steady means to acquire necessities to survive. This includes material acquisitions that serve interest and entertainment. Threats to our income and careers attack this significant building block in the pyramid. We then fixate and fight to preserve our possessions which derails our maturation and progress in personal, emotional, and spiritual development. Once security needs are fulfilled, we search for identity through our relationships. We desire to belong, have family, establish a supportive interactive community and experience love.

We simultaneously need to maintain independence and a strong sense of self, and not be consumed by strictly our social identity. Our core values mature through interpersonal relationships and a healthy sense of self. This state of being, combined with strong social ties, is proven as our healthies psychological state. Through these connections we desire praise, status, affirmation and recognition for our diligent and ongoing efforts as healthcare providers. Lastly, as we grant and receive empathetic acknowledgment of our human frailty, find our spiritual path, and separate ourselves from petty conflicts and narcissistic obsessions, we may achieve self-actualization. Transitioning between the last two levels of the pyramid, we experience a freedom from the strain of toxic conflict and hold reverent the interconnection and commonality of the human need for fulfillment. Our efforts evolve from self-preservation to providing for the needs and interests of the community of humanity.

Conflict develops as a manifestation of our perceptions and positions, claiming our need for fulfillment, which contrasts with another person's needs and interests. Our lives are constantly balancing our desire for personal and professional acceptance and admiration, poised against distributive demands from people with whom we interact. Conflict occurs through claimed positions and interests and assumes an opponent's claim can only be achieved by devaluing and dismissing our rights to our perceived rewards. We attribute the other parties needs as an attempt to exert superiority, control, and power over us, and respond with escalating resistance and deepening fixation, driven toward a dominant and winning posture over this adversary.

Conflict has many roots, and there are many theories to explain its origins. Conflict is expressed as a basic human instinct, evolving from competition for resources and power, developed as integral within the structure of the societies and institutions. Conflict is nurtured from the inevitable struggle defined by race and socio-economic status that separates persons into unique cultures. When we understand the motivation behind conflict behavior, we are suited to envision selective and effective approaches to handling conflict. The wheel of conflict, as described by Professor Bernie Mayer, illustrates conflict as a derivative of human needs. People engage in conflict to fulfill unsatisfied needs that are inconsistent with those of others. Until the needs and interests are addressed in some way, conflict persists. Expression of those needs during conflict is affected by the method of interpersonal communication, emotive expressions, fundamental individualized values and the context defining the interaction between opposing parties. In addition, history and future potential relationships significantly influence the nature of the dispute.

Parties always assume they communicate clearly and honestly, however conflict escalation proves that assumption is false. Individuals are sure that opponents have the same information and choose to obstruct our access to needs and interests, attributing this to devious and bad behavior instead of the imperfections of human communication. As Dr. Mayer points out 'People often rely on inaccurate or incomplete perceptions, tend to form stereotypes, and carry into their communications conclusions drawn from former interactions or experiences. They are also inclined to try to solve problems before they understand them. The greater the duress a person is under, the harder it is for him or her to communicate.'

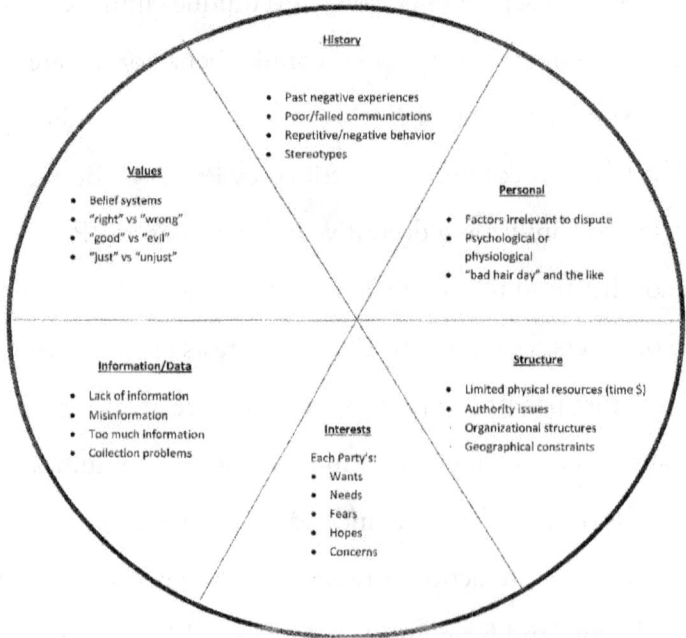

History
- Past negative experiences
- Poor/failed communications
- Repetitive/negative behavior
- Stereotypes

Values
- Belief systems
- "right" vs "wrong"
- "good" vs "evil"
- "just" vs "unjust"

Personal
- Factors irrelevant to dispute
- Psychological or physiological
- "bad hair day" and the like

Information/Data
- Lack of information
- Misinformation
- Too much information
- Collection problems

Structure
- Limited physical resources (time $)
- Authority issues
- Organizational structures
- Geographical constraints

Interests
Each Party's:
- Wants
- Needs
- Fears
- Hopes
- Concerns

Wheel of Conflict

Usually emotions drive behavior and are frequently used as an expression of power during a dispute. Anger, rage, and demanding positions contribute to the perseverance that allows opponents to meet the challenges of a conflict. The power behind these displays functions to suppress fears threatening an individual's sense of righteousness and self-worth. During conflict management, opponents are given the opportunity to express their emotional energy to a receptive audience who listens with understanding and empathy, providing both catharsis and often a pathway toward resolution. However, venting frustration is often tainted with accusations and challenges toward the opponent, resulting in escalation of the dispute. Thus dialogue which establishes a safe and non-threatening environment for all parties to decompress their emotions, usually with a skilled third party directing the conversation, is an effective tool during discovery and resolution of conflict behavior.

Disputes emanate from individualized value systems, or beliefs in what is important, what is right or wrong, and what is good or evil. These principals govern our lives, and conflicts developing from alternative value systems are often intractable and escalate over time. Since people identify with core beliefs, when these are attacked, the assault threatens both identity and integrity. By remaining in the conflict, a person might view themselves as honorable and virtuous while dehumanizing their opponent who embodies evil, malicious, and dangerous claims. Though values instigate and perpetuate disputes, finding commonality in value systems is quite effective at restraining opponents and moving toward negotiated compromise. Recognizing when values are an important issue in the conflict is a critical step toward constructive discourse and potential resolution. A conversation that expresses personal values without attacking opposing views invites acceptance and collaboration.

The structure in which a dispute is addressed has significant impact on potential resolution. In facilitated and mediated discussion, compatible interests steer people toward a cooperative consideration for resolution. However, if the structure of communication is adversarial, exemplified by the litigation process, conflict is often exacerbated. Although litigation does achieve a decisive outcome, as a structural framework for conflict resolution, opponents experience greater antipathy and malice toward their opponent in this win-lose scenario.

Disputes must be understood while considering the historical relationship of opponents. History provides the momentum for the development of conflict. As individuals or social groups, even minor disputes are exacerbated if past interaction was competitive and distributional, where only victors and defeated existed after conflicts were settled. When a productive future relationship can be envisioned by the parties, collaboration on options to resolve disputes are effectively introduced by both opponents and the facilitators managing the conversation. The alternatives are often expressed when the structure of the conversation includes a mediated framework that interprets claims as opportunities for conflict resolution.

Needs according to Maslow are very different than interests. Accordingly, interests are considered transient and situational whereas needs are basic human requirements. Upon consideration, most disputes arise over interest that diverge between parties. Moore suggests three types of interests: substantive (concerns about tangible benefits), procedural (concerns about a process for interacting, communicating, or decision making), and psychological (concerns about how one is treated, respected, or acknowledged). These may be short-term or long-term interests, individual or group interests, outcome-based or process interests, and conscious vs unconscious interests. A third party, such as a facilitator, must establish the type of the opponent's interests during conflict management, concentrating on similar mutually beneficial interests to establish a common definition such that perception between adversaries is aligned. When opponents are assisted at constructive expression of their interests and willing to extend an empathetic consideration to their adversaries, we are best prepared to reveal integrative and collaborative solutions to most conflicts.

In contrast, actual needs that define core identity must be achieved by both parties to preserve their sense of self and role in their own world. We can redefine Maslow's pyramid as the needs for meaning, community, intimacy, and autonomy. In some situations, persons who resist conflict resolution desire to stay engaged in the dispute, for it functions as a great source of meaning for these individuals. In addition, dispute management that fails to consider a person's identity within their group or social structure is doomed to fail. Persons, and entire groups for that matter, are exceedingly protective of their social identity from which Moore explains, 'their sense of personal security, belonging, and autonomy will flow.' Identity conflicts are high stakes conflicts and traditional application of demanding legal rules are often inadequate to address the underlying needs and emotions of the individual. A disaffected opponent attributes their ultimate position to the malice of their superior and refuses to psychologically accept a subordinate power position. Any successful compromise must weigh these value-based interests when attempting to achieve long term peaceful solutions.

In attribution theory, people strive to understand the causes of events around them, particularly other people's behavior, because accurate understanding of these causes helps people make appropriate and adaptive responses to those events creating conflict. This social psychology theory maintains we become reflexively angry and experience an impulse to strike back when presented with opposing positions threatening our claims. We then interpret opposition behavior as either the core maladaptive traits and values of the individual, or as Heider's work describes, their dispositions (such as their personality traits, attitudes, or abilities). On occasion we attribute the contrary behavior of others to the external circumstances affecting their actions, assuming their personality traits have fundamentally benevolent intentions. The distinction is important as the more we perceive a negative action to be the intended result of someone's behavior, the more we attribute their behavior to malignant disposition. Research indicates that when individuals attribute other people's behavior to dispositional narcissism, they are ignoring contrary information that supports the other's circumstances affecting the opponents claims and positions. In contrast, we usually reject our own maladaptive or self-serving behavior as a matter of circumstance, while deceiving ourselves and rejecting the fact that our own dispositions may be the cause of the conflict. This is referred to as the actor-observer bias.

The bias perception extends to group dynamic behavior as we frequently attribute an out-group member's negative behavior to the person's defects of character or disposition while considering the mis-behavior of our own group member caused from circumstances and not defects in their pristine character traits. This intergroup attributional bias has significant perceptual influence during disputes over conflicting interests or in any long-standing conflict, pitting social groups against each other. As an example in healthcare, a disaffected and embarrassed individual nurse recruits a nursing cadre to support his maligning views of a physician, attributing the physician's claiming demands as a personality defect. The nurse attributes the provider's actions as a reflection of a difficult and disruptive individual, while dismissing circumstances that the provider might perceive as a critical threat to her patient's well-being. The ensuing conflict between individuals and the larger group personality escalates with polar and defensive adverse positions and communication between this provider and the entire nursing contingent subsequently deteriorates, threatening quality of care.

As we fight our opponent, we become entrapped by the conflict itself. Our continued position and involvement in a dispute is justified by our past involvement and we cannot "let go" and resolve the issue. People who believe they are grievously injured are bitterly antagonistic and become irrationally committed to a fight. It is exceedingly difficult to disengage and to admit our position was either wrong or not worth the passion placed in the adversarial dispute. As the stakes of a conflict rise, such as in a tort claim, entrapment plays an important role in decision making and risk assessment by both plaintiffs and defendants. Both sides assert their rights and positions are the only viable conclusion a reasonable judge or jury could make. There is a mistaken tendency to dismiss the opponents position as frivolous and wrong with an actor-observer bias. Priest and Klein demonstrated that the plaintiff in such an action actually fare much worse than the defendant in this prediction game. In an attempt to circumvent extreme positions and influence an exchange to resolve disputes, negotiation theorists pay attention to the perceptual and behavioral reactions evolving during an increasingly intense and competitive bargaining process. Strategies and definitions of "winning" a dispute are often more concerned with avoiding loss than achieving some gain over their opponent. In fact, the avoidance of loss is pursued more vigorously than the prospect of gain. In medical malpractice cases we witness loss aversion frequently as the defendant provider aggressively defends a weak medical decision or action rather than settle, because the prospect of a large uncertain loss (losing the case) is more acceptable than the knowledge of a small, certain one (settling and allowing the patient to successfully claim the provider did something wrong).

Another phenomenon frequently observed is that of reactive devaluation. Here, one party dismisses a compromise proposal when its offered by the other disputing party, but the same proposal offered by a neutral third party is accepted. Providers will reject the proposal from a plaintiff lawyer but accept a similar compromise from a third party neutral mediator.

Psychologists and academics Felstiner, Abel, and Sarat consider personal reactions to conflict influenced by the social and cultural contexts surrounding a dispute. Conflict management strategies are influenced by cultural acceptance. In some cultures, indicative of Western Anglo-American individualism, conflict avoidance is regarded as negative, however in Asian cultures this strategy is an honorable way to ensure that no opponent loses face during the dispute. Similarly, silence is assumed to be an avoiding behavior but culturally utilized as an effective strategy to mitigate harm caused by the conflict. These authors also describe the process of turning a problem into a dispute as 'naming, blaming, and claiming', where a robust conflict progresses through each stage, gaining emotive and value-based positional demands by both sides.

Social constructionists query how and why people perceive and value the same experience differently and, in this difference, consider an action or perspective as contrary to their needs and interests. Once a person or group considers an event or action as injurious and devaluating, they 'name' the dispute and the opponent. This is a critical transformation and creates the perceived grievance. This can only occur when a person attributes an injury to the fault of another individual or group. Fault is by definition a violation of what should be a normal action or behavior and also assumes the misstep and bad action has some form of remedy. The transformation from perceived injurious experience to grievance is 'blaming.' When the remedy is demanded by a party, this person is 'claiming' resolution only by accomplishing the remedial action. If that claim is rejected by an opponent, the dispute occurs.

Disputes are therefore subjective, reactive, complicated, and incomplete as the desired remedy rarely addresses the emotional turmoil or psychological impact inferred by the initial named event. As a disputant searches for social support, often counseled by persons who are only trained in distributional justice such as lawyers, the disputant is empowered and transforms their perspective of the event, attributing the behavior of the opposing party as an act of purposeful bad faith. These are all emotive considerations. As they change, the dispute and process to resolve the issues are unstable. The prevailing ideology defining civil litigation is support for the individual's sense of entitlement, to enjoy certain experiences and be free from others. Attribution errors play a critical role in the progression of conflict positioning.

Healthcare providers are often astonished during litigation that a former patient and their family, people the provider believed were kind and appreciated the provider's dedicated efforts, morphed into hostile maligning plaintiffs. This should be no surprise as advocates for the plaintiffs utilize the instability of emotive valuation to their benefit, stirring the embers of discontent and resentment by converting an action perceived as "malpractice" into an act of bad faith purposefully committed and thereby victimizing the patient. The family, by loss of enjoyment of the healthy patient, exerts a derivative claim against the provider. Pursuing justice through litigation further ensures a reactive defensive polar position by all parties. As we shall discuss, that is contrary to the philosophical approaches of transformative dispute resolution.

To further understanding conflict evolution, we consider McFarland's summary of reactive posturing as the typologies and conflict styles individuals assume as their major strategy when faced with dispute. These are avoidance or yielding, lowering ones expectations or demands by accommodating, responding with assertive contending or competitive strategies, and collaborative interests-based approaches with problem solving to discover expanded resources for settlement. An individual's orientation toward managing conflict can be measured using the Briggs-Mayer psychological survey or the Thomas-Kilmann Instrument (TKI). These questioners measure tactics people commonly employ when faced with a conflict. The style they choose will have both advantages and disadvantages in certain circumstances. For instance, avoiding conflict is not usually a good tactical move but when used strategically, for example to create a delay in negotiations, it may be quite effective. For protracted issues, avoidance is unwise.

Not uncommonly in healthcare, avoidance occurs when the hierarchical system supports powerful providers whose conflict behavior harasses perceived subordinates. As an example, a nurse who always avoids conflict even when in the right, is subverting her profession's goal of ensuring quality healthcare delivery. These situations must not prevail. Avoidance occurs due to fear, lack of knowledge of management process, absence of interdependent interests, indifference to the issues in the dispute, or belief that an agreement is not possible and further conflict is not desirable. Persons who use this tactic may decide to pursue their interests independently, trying to limit their interaction with the opponent. Not uncommonly, people or groups repeatedly defeated frequently withdraw and avoid disputes just to preserve their continued survival, anticipating defeat is inevitable. The psychological impact of lost hope for improved situation is significant.

As an alternative, accommodation occurs when one party agrees to meet the interests of their opponent at their own expense. One side may accommodate in a resolution and sacrifice its own interests to maintain a future relationship with the other, choosing to cooperate and concede and ensure an amicable outcome. Unfortunately some parties accommodate because they lack power or authority over their opponent and revert to a passive posturing during dispute negotiations. When one parties goal is to ease the tension of conflict by acquiescing important needs just to preserve harmony and relationships, the outcome should reward the yielding party with some long-term benefit. Of course accommodating works well when one is in the wrong or if the issue is significantly more important to the other party and one side chooses to build goodwill. However, someone who routinely accommodates will be victimized by more powerful opponents.

The polar extreme uses the competing style which is usually a less than optimal approach to conflict resolution. This is the classic distributive model in which the goal is to "win" at all costs. Litigation in front of judge or jury requires this behavior. The parties are positional, demanding, assertive, and avoid cooperation. The competing style uses intimidation and coercion to accomplish its own goals. In hierarchical systems like healthcare, someone forcing resolution by asserting rank, status or privilege is both competitive and often a high conflict personality typology.

Theoretically the style assumes that one party is demanding to achieve benefits only for themselves, however when a critical issue arises and a party with both authority and responsibility must decide and act quickly, even if the course of action is unpopular, the competing style must be employed. Careful application of the competing style by a senior medical team provider will avoid disempowered colleagues, nurses and technicians. When the team must accept an unwavering authoritarian dictatorship, this ultimately results in disaffected individuals whose compromised morale interrupts the mission to provide quality patient care.

Compromising style in negotiating and bargaining results in

resolution only after concessions are offered by both parties. This occurs when opponents do not believe that competition viewed as a win-lose situation, as offered through the court system, will see them prevail. They also reject a win-win solution which requires trust and collaboration as even a possibility. Their interests seem incompatible and disparate from their opponent. The parties do not trust each other enough to enter into joint problem solving for mutual gain. Through compromise, parties attempt to meet most of their needs, dividing and sharing limited resources. Generally both sides have equal authority and power in the negotiation, so a forced solution is not possible. Although this tactic can be useful in temporary settlements, it is best reserved when issues are not extremely important to either party. It is unlikely that peace will be preserved as parties required to concede significant positions become cynical and will undermine the settlement, returning with emotional and value-based convictions to dominate the opponent in future disputes. Parties in litigation who reach a negotiated settlement, such as a medical malpractice case, typically find their advocates encouraging this style, assuming that a monetary settlement is an adequate compromise. The misperception that one party receiving money to resolve the claim is balanced by the promise to end the dispute and keep the payment confidential does not resolve the underlying conflict. This compromised style does not address the emotional and value convictions of either party, thus both sides retain the anger and resentment brought by the litigation. This is a psychologically unhealthy result for either plaintiff patient or defendant provider.

In general, the discipline of dispute resolution advocates for interest-based negotiation between opponents, assuming that the competition and compromise models only achieve settlement by the division of fixed resources. In contrast, interest-based techniques fundamentally use dialogue, active listening and inquisition to expose both needs and interests. As Gerardi points out, 'listening is typically restricted to information needed to move through the day and is rarely done at a level that enables understanding of a situation where there may be collaboration.' The interest-based process predicts that when parties interact empathetically they will collaborate on alternative options that increase the possibility and diversity of solutions to any problem. In essence, the effort tries to expand the range of possibilities resolving all issues so that the needs of the parties are considered and achieved.

Third-party intermediaries, such as mediators, are particularly effective when skilled at these techniques, encouraging trust between conflicting individuals who view their success as interdependent. The parties understand that solutions that ensure their opponents achieve their goals have the greatest chance of mutual adoption. People pursue this approach when they are significantly invested in a mutually satisfactory outcome, recognizing that the cost of impasse is too great, and they wish to maintain a respectful and productive future relationship. Collaborating on problems causing disputes is effective problem solving and when utilized objectively, results in institutional improvement and superior quality objectives. Healthcare organizations who employ active engagement of conflict identification and resolution are superior in medical delivery models. The interest-based style is challenging since collaborating involves significant individual assertiveness and cooperation, listening to and understanding alternative perspectives, then merging new insights into functional solutions. True integrative problem solving relies upon trusting the other party to act in good faith and with one's interests at heart.

Trust can be defined in several ways. A fundamentally calculus-based trust occurs when parties believe that their opponent will act in a consistent way and do what they promised. This trust assumes that fear of retribution against a defaulting party maintains the trust, so by extending a reserved calculus-based trust, the granting party anticipates some negotiated reward. Individuals want to be considered trustworthy and recognize the threat to their reputation and subsequent social and professional consequences if they break the trust.

In contrast, identity-based trust is a committed trust where individuals act with complete confidence that another person will represent their interests as they would for themselves. Thus, each person behaves seamlessly as one individual, with the highest regard for the benefit of their colleague and friend. To accomplish identity-based trust, the values, beliefs and moral principles are co-joined and enmeshed and each individual is confident their trust mate will act exactly as they would during external negotiations. Empathy is strongest in this group. Because of the deep-seated nature of the interpersonal commitment, conflicts arising in identity-based relationships are often difficult to repair.

As healthcare providers we should recognize the differential of trust expectations with our patients and their family. We perform our duties and assume we are establishing a calculus-based trust of practical promises with our patient. The patient however is granting us the most intimate access to their body and psyches and views the relationship with implicit identity-based trust. Therefore, when conflicts arise, the provider's intellectual management of the dispute is usually not enough to re-establish trust, satisfaction and resolution for the patient and family. An effective method of repairing the patients broken identity-based trust is communication focusing on shared common goals and values. Reiterating that as providers we desire the same solution as the patient, share identical concerns, interests and needs for their care and that our goal is always to optimize patient safety and mitigate any further physical or emotional damage following an unexpected result. Working with the patient and family and letting them be party to a collaborative problem-solving methodology which prevents future misunderstandings, supports reestablished trust and resolution through an integrative approach.

Mayer provides insight into the dynamics of conflict analysis by opposing parties and maintains that resolution occurs when they experience acceptable levels of solutions in cognitive, emotional, and behavioral dimensions. Understanding the interests and needs of each opponent in terms of acceptable resolution must discover, then achieve, these dimensional objectives. To confound the settlement process, as a conflict emerges and matures, individual's goals and objectives often change over time. In principal, opponents will only accept resolution when they perceive their key issues are addressed and view the conflict as part of their past, and not their future. Resolution in the cognitive dimension is usually the most difficult, as opponents are often tenaciously resistant to change their perceptions about a conflict. These beliefs are often the cornerstone of a person's sense of stability and order, and the conflict threatens their self-perception and self-conceived intrinsic value to their world.

Often, a willingness to resolve a conflict requires changing their views of a situation and admitting they were wrong. Many people refuse to concede this position. Although difficult to reach, when these cognitive hurdles are overcome, we see profound position changes helping to resolve the conflict state. Emotional resolution is also challenging as disputants behaviors mirror their emotional conviction to an argument. Devaluation of the emotional impact of an argument by the opposition breeds contempt and hostility. Only true empathy can resolve emotional turmoil. When disputants accept through empathy the value within their opponents perception, they change their essential view of their adversary. The conflict then loses intrinsic value and committed energy and emotional resolution is possible.

A professional intervening to assist these parties addresses the three dimensions of resolution by using a variety of healing and confidence building activities which force parties to reevaluate their views. As an example, skills utilized for cognitive resolution include creation of cognitive dissonance followed by successive reframing of the conflict. Cognitive dissonance results as the values or positions held by an individual come into conflict with each other, forcing some level of change in that person's belief system. The technique of reframing attempts to redefine how the conflict is perceived through the narrative presentation, acknowledging but neutralizing extreme emotional positions, thereby discovering options for resolution. The emotional dimension of resolution involves releasing both the feelings and the emotional energy each party contribute to the fight. This only occurs when the dedicated intensity and volatility of demonstrative turbulence by adversaries is abandon. Disputants often achieve a sense of emotional closure just by feeling comfortable and less anxious about the dispute. Unfortunately, they may rebound into heated argument when interaction with their adversaries reawaken unpleasant feelings.

Behavioral resolution to disputes are exemplified by agreements, contracts and negotiated settlements. Although these may resolve the current dispute, when this settlement involves distributional negotiations or awards, emotional and cognitive conflict remain. The parties will never reestablish a long-term trusting, empathetic or compassionate relationship. Actual complete resolution only occurs when cognitive, emotional and behavioral resolution is accomplished. Research has found that apology and forgiveness are important aspects for comprehensive dispute settlements when these are expressed honestly. Forgiveness by a party victimized by an offender allows them to release the passionate energy of anger that is fueling the dispute. With this act, a victim humanizes their adversary, establishing empathy between opponents, and comes closer to resolving the conflict strangling their ascent of Maslow's pyramid.

Disputes become more difficult when parties defending a moral and value-based position refuse to negotiate, compromise or collaborate on any solutions. This is frustrating when dispute resolution is practical and mutually beneficial. The rights-based model of resolution is the foundation of the judicial system. In this distributional model, individual's claims assume they are entitled to rights that are oppressed by their adversaries' position. Conflict resolution using alternative means to litigation in rights-based claims are very challenging, requiring significant empathetic understanding and capitulation by parties at moral odds with each other.

Collaborating on solutions is often a remote possibility. Resource based disputes occur over fixed assets or rights to those assets, such as a provider groups right to a population insured by a third-party carrier. These disputes are not morally inspired so usually easier to define. Although emotional commitment to a dispute can be significant, usually these type of disputes respond to interest-based negotiations and stimulate potential templates for conflict settlement. Resource-based disputes can quickly devolve into identity-based arguments when either party believes they are entitled or deserve something more than their opponent. The resultant lawsuit then adopts language of moral principal and outrage, claiming value based upon compromise of identity-based transgressions, while really attempting to maximize a resource-based resolution (money for the plaintiff).

Protracted conflicts are almost always identity-based with attribution errors between parties. Each side claims the moral imperative not to settle because the opposite sides transgression is a matter of character flaws and not because of a disagreement or action that occurred in this situation. Positions are maintained because of

46

'moral principal' by one or both parties. As Riskin notes, tactics taught and utilized by lawyers 'differ radically from that which a mediator must use.' He confirms that the lawyers guiding principles are distributional success between adversaries where only one party can win, and that disputes only conclude through judgment by an authoritative individual who applies fixed general rules of law.

The theoretical basis of litigation in an adjudicative model justifies the opinion that conflict is best resolved in the court system, reinforcing this assumption by asserting that judicial decisions are the only effective means to establish right vs. wrong, define what is desirable or undesirable, and to bring justice to an injustice compromising society. Legal proceedings are constant and reproducible. First, information is gathered in order to substantiate a particular version of events, so even when confounding information weakens the assertion, that information is often discarded or ignored. Evidence is generated to enhance the perspective of this rights-based argument, dismissing information that does not support the argument as irrelevant. The advocates position will present information as evidence and assert it factual and beyond reproach, compelling a decision to favor her argument over the opponents claims.

Litigation is a zero-sum model described by game theory with the side representing the most complete and well-constructed argument is awarded the victory. During information gathering (discovery), knowledge is not shared, it is gathered and then used selectively to advance ones position over the opponent, zealously advocating rights based and resource-based claims. Lawyers reframe a dispute to support their position by either narrowing or broadening facts in a structural paradigm recognized by the litigation model for civil claims. Advocates frequently alternatively define actual facts and stories to fit their narrative, viewing solutions only as win-lose propositions. By reiterating their tale of selective and massaged truths, presenting embellished and distorted charges for public consumption, the lawyer attempts to leverage social condemnation against the opponent, seeking to prejudice and influence, while maintaining a high monetary value to the claim. These tactics try to extract concession from opponents fearing social castigation or overwhelmed with litigation fatigue. Healthcare providers with insurance covering their acts or omissions are perfect fodder for aggressive plaintiff litigators.

As Menkel-Meadow points out, even when a client tells a broad and robust story, the lawyer will narrow the version to fit into a recognizable sound bite that can justify a claim for remediation. The lawyer enters the negotiation demanding a progressively focused solution requiring compensation. This is the only approach he will follow mirroring what he will ask the court to award in damages should the case proceed to trial. Most lawsuits in negotiation, as they would be at trial, quickly convert to zero sum, win-lose outcomes in which money is considered the only remedial cure. Since negotiation is about compromise, both sides concede something in order to settle the dispute. For instance, in a medical malpractice case, the healthcare provider concedes money even while rejecting the assumption of blame or guilt. Unfortunately she must understand the implication of settling a case for monetary damages, as publication in the national practitioner database and possible refusal of privileges during a credentialing investigation, do consider a settlement synonymous with the commission of a malpractice act. Since the patient turned victim receives money as the only reward, they never get an apology, explanation, or assurance that the system is safer. In fact, only lawyers are satisfied in these cases. Any provider participating in a settlement conference is warned that opposing arguments will shift the judge and jury position, even when inaccurate, because the opposing counsel is "an excellent trial lawyer."

Healthcare providers learn that inaccurate arguments made persuasively using "reptile tactics" play on the inherent fears of jurors. A plaintiff's lawyer argues that a provider's accused error is a character flaw of the practitioner and will be repeated, possibly hurting someone close to the juror. Only by finding the provider liable will she be held accountable. Providers hear that juries are "funny animals and unpredictable" and therefore a settlement is better for everyone. As healthcare practitioners, we cringe at the grey area of legal processes and find the illogical and subjective decision-making exercise extremely frustrating. We reject methods and conclusions that are not based on facts analyzed using the scientific method. Practitioners are lost in the sea of litigation treachery that advocates perception over truth. As a defendant, the provider will find his recitation of facts and defenses interpreted as positional claiming and emotionally reactive. Nearly always, a logical conclusion would demonstrate that unanticipated outcomes are not errors of omission or commission, but unfortunate consequences of imperfect scientific application. The actual facts are rejected by the provider's opponent, even when impartially represented by independent experts. Finally, the lay press narrative is often established and reiterated by godless plaintiff's attorneys regurgitating their version of an opaque truth.

Chapter Three

The Problem for Providers

Healthcare providers, each with their own perspective on both problem relevance and solution priorities, naturally interact in an environment defined by incongruity, where the complex puzzle pieces in case management either don't fit together or our way of solving the problem is perceived alternatively or adversely by our colleague's approach to the case. Our expectation diverges from reality and we claim our rights in patient care decision-making authority. As we demand and claim or take a positional rights-based approach to conflict, we create a divisive dichotomy rejecting collaborative teamwork needed to secure optimal outcome. This dispositional approach automatically assumes there is a winner and loser in every conversation and decision, and this is the essence of dysfunctional communication in healthcare.

The natural defensive response from our opponent, who themselves are concerned about respect, reputation, professional autonomy or even liability, is in fact to do the same; name the issue and claim the position or make demands that let them "win" in the conversation. As each side moves away from a solution, respecting both opinions equally, the instinct is to consider the entire relationship as adversarial and minimize current and future communication. This shuts off the free flow of information and education so critical to patient care delivery. Adversarial confrontations that yields winners and losers is so ingrained in the execution of medical care delivery that many believe there are no alternatives to these tactics. With the constantly evolving micro-management of healthcare delivery by business and federal entities, the rules and regulations often create impediments to actual patient treatment and we realize we must negotiate just to practice good medicine.

Practitioners are programmed to be competitive, positional and want to win. Adversarial methods of negotiation with positional demands derive from our instinctual drive for self-protection. Our amygdala-controlled reflex responds to threats, assuming they herald our demise. Control becomes a matter of defense. Fearing brutality and defeat, whether physical, personal or professional, the provider alleviates anxiety by outmaneuvering and destroying today's enemy. Civility may be abandoned. Parties involved in an adversarial, high-stakes dispute often become obsessed with victory over their contenders. Whether an event is a care management opinion, an actual malpractice issue, conflict between hospital departments, or an internal staff dispute at the health care clinic, each side sets its objectives and gauges its progress by conquering the other side. The "other's" perspective and their power to influence our behavior becomes our adversary.

Conflict does become a matter of obsession as time, costs, and distractions accumulate for each side. Stake holder parties become convinced that their professional futures can only be guaranteed by winning the day, and equally they must destroy their opponent. But an interesting metamorphosis occurs when we are convinced that we are 'right'. Logic cedes to psychological trickery. We obsess in our alternative reality, ignoring facts and refusing to consider we maybe misinformed. We are self-convinced of distorted objectivity and label any error of our doing as a matter of subjective opinion. The time, effort and commitment invested into this distortion is not easily abandon. Preventative attention and objective consideration of all stake holder's perspectives and interests, before arriving at conclusions, will prevent sliding into a self-righteous position, a very lonely place indeed. We often fail to account for the multiple personalities involved in the conversation, each exponentially impacting every problem. Whether those involved are physician and nurse, patient and clinician, or administrator and staff member, there are a myriad of ways for players to get mired in recalcitrant perceptions when assessing an identical problem. Once parties adopt a line of thinking, they can become allegiant to it. The interchange then becomes passionate as each advocate and defend their principles. Conflict is a process of polarization and when two people are in an argument, they characteristically migrate to opposite sides of the issue. They fortify their own positions, zealously overstating their case, and ignore information that does not conform to their thinking. As the conflict escalates, they become more resolute in defending their position and destroying their opponent. Everything the other side does is woven into the story of who, not what, is right or wrong. Conflict is also a process of simplification. We ignore the reasons, justifications, viewpoints, and concerns of the other side. Our opponent's position is without merit and ours is valid. Our thinking is reduced to clear-cut terms and we are blind to the weaknesses of our own shortcomings and fantasized reality. Bad conflict is a bitter distraction, is costly, and can be destructive, especially when negotiating critical decisions regarding health care. Bad conflict is conducted in an adversarial manner in which defeating or even destroying the other side becomes more important than solving the presenting problem. Achieving an integrated viewpoint is essential with health care negotiation and the conflict resolution process.

As we begin to observe and understand conflict, we can make choices about both substance and process. We can learn from conflict. Good conflict effectively exposes problems, generates creativity, and develops solutions not previously considered. Discussion is conducted in a respectful manner, focused on the problem and not the individual, and it follows a mutually accepted structure. Conflict discourse is a vehicle to assist with introspection, understand the people we work with, and define our common objectives and interests. Complexity theory defines health care as an interconnected complex organism. When any individual exchange malfunctions the entire organic machine devolves, is less efficient and loses effective direction. As professionals we known that common and shared responsibility fosters shared methodology and remedies. Individuals who constructively frame conflict as a positive exchange encourage respectful expression and acknowledgment of differences, and during subsequent bargaining, all legitimate concerns are considered.

Characteristically, greater numbers of parties involved in, and affected by a decision, results in exponentially more positional claims in a conflict. The stakes differ considerably for the many people involved. Those stakes are measured in terms of professional responsibility, legal or financial liability, personal pride, quality of life, time, pain, and personal stress. Now, add competition and divergent interests by competing professions and institutions, each wielding different amounts of power and status, and disruptive acrimonious conflict becomes a quagmire for the healthcare provider. We see this constantly where there are turf war issues and challenges in competence as the youth in training mature their own knowledge and experience.

Given the extraordinary interdependence of health care services, distributive conflict demands and its adversarial consequences put pressure on the entire system. When the most incendiary ingredients are flung into this mix, conflict behavior is ugly and frightening. Mistrust, lies, deception, and malicious actions breed suspicion and aggression. Manipulation, fear, hostility, and counterstrategies insert a dynamic that appears insurmountable to interrupt. As emotions fuel thinking and behavior, each side assumes a battle position. The outrageous acts of one side goad and justify malcontent from the opposite camp. Eventually, people lose sight of the original issues and the impact resolution might have on professional practice. The conflict assumes an independent dark life force. Anyone who opposes our cause is "the enemy." Vanquishing the enemy portends a virtue unto itself, propelling the battle mission into a matter of personal pride and survival. The true cost of this bad conflict inflicts wounds far deeper than merely an expensive legal bill, lost time, or frazzled emotions. It starves one's soul.

For the managed care organization, nursing department, or medical practice, the real costs of unresolved conflict are the combined losses for staff members in terms of morale, wellbeing and the dispute's effect on the quality of delivered medical attention. Infighting among coalition members results in lost services and support for the patient. Metrix measuring adverse patient outcomes, diminished satisfaction, professional turnover, malpractice litigation and provider burn out, all correlate with the intensity of dispositional animosity prevalent in the institution and clinic. For the patient, a breakdown in communication with providers causes feelings of vulnerability and anxiety over interrupted care. These negatively impact the health status of the patient. One caustic example is a medical group maligning the care or surgical results of their competitor, generating complaints to medical boards and causing malpractice litigation between clinicians and surgeons. Professional practices are devastated by these unethical disputes and disaster for the provider is guaranteed.

Paradoxically, the true winners in the healthcare marketplace are learning that the best way to ensure their survival is by finding new strategies to collaborate, partner, and inspire each other's creativity. Joint ventures, interoperable technologies, consolidations, and mergers, even though difficult to galvanize, provide a protective position of strength in the face of rapid and volatile change. Working through the anger and frustration of resistance in the system is an abhorrent but necessary process. When we progress from angry, venting and demanding ultimatums to active listening, learning, and collaborative exploration, we usually arrive with superior resolution through a symbiotic agreement and options that support our initial intent.

Chapter Four

Skills, strategies and key concepts for managing disputes involving the healthcare team members

Dialogue – The operational definition of effective conflict communication is best quoted by Boehm: 'in dialogue this can be experienced both individually and collectively. Each listener is able to reflect back to each speaker, and to the rest of the group, a view of some of the assumptions and unspoken implications of what is being expressed along with that which is being avoided.' The relationship of self to the group asserts 'it creates the opportunity for each participant to examine the preconceptions, prejudices and the characteristic patterns that lie behind his or her thoughts, opinions, beliefs and feelings, along with the roles he or she tends habitually to play... it offers an opportunity to share these insights.' Furthermore dialogue itself 'is not concerned with deliberately trying to alter or change behavior, nor to get the participants to move toward a predetermined goal.' Instead, dialogue as a structured discourse appreciates a resultant change in perspective that manifests through individual action. The experience expands perspectives and considers alternatives, not as threats, but possibilities for a peaceful and prosperous future.

Achieving effective dialogue is a quite interesting technique. Effective dialogue begins by quieting prejudice and bias between parties. Effective dialogue requires active listening, empathy, and the ability to discount one's own belief system based upon normative cultural values, while granting authority and permission for an alternative viewpoint to interpret the same facts and situation that created the dispute. Effective dialogue is learning and requires receptive interpretation of disputed issues by alternative sources, suspending our potentially limited positional opinions while not abandoning our own committed interests. We must be willing to share our understanding of reality. In essence, effective dialogue requires all parties to express self-interests but accept an alternative conclusion once credence and authority are granted to another's views. Parties in conflict exposed to well-constructed dialogue framework will more likely behave civilly and act professionally for the greater good. To caution, any technique that assumes that self-interest will not trump communal resolution in societies that celebrate personal power, material possessions, and authoritative rule, will be difficult and strain our resolve. Maintaining effective dialogue is challenging as those in power generally relish and protect the perception of power. We live in a culture of individualism that maintains a symbiotic cohabitation with both social and cultural order by individuals who share the same central theme. Therefore entrenched perspectives will contest the value of effective discourse and dialogue. Nevertheless, it is noble and worthy to actualize an open integrative mind, disregard materialism, and strive for the greater cause of peace and shared prosperity.

Negotiation strategies: Positional Bargaining vs Integrative negotiation

To begin, accept the intrinsic value in conflict. When professional disputes are normalized and accepted, the problems are simply issues requiring a solution, stimulating a potentially creative aspect of our work. Identification and naming the issues should be encouraged. Eliminating apprehension or fear and voicing a concern is an important regulator in health care. If a nurse believes an inappropriate medication is being prescribed, flagging the problem will benefit the patient, the provider who ordered the medication, and the health system in which the problem occurs. The interchange can be constructive only if the nurse is aware of a protected method to question an order, without fear of retribution or demeaning accusation by the prescribing author. From a patient safety perspective, encouraging proactive expressions of concern establishes an important layer of protection.

When only one party wants to find a solution, the conflict is likely to continue. People must be ready to settle their dispute. Through investigative conversation and discussion, any vengeful antagonism must be acknowledged, but adverse feelings must be quelled in order to consider an agreeable compromise. In so doing, remember that saving face and avoiding embarrassment to either party is critical to conclude any dispute. Conflict is often accompanied by a story, a narrative. Parties in dispute have a set of stories that line up with their version of the "facts." To listen to your opponent is not the same as agreeing to their theory. An open mind will look for truths and any validity to what the other person is saying. Finding common ground is a process of joint discovery, working together to develop options for settlement. An option might be a compromise. It could be an exchange, an acknowledgment of differences or an apology. In the process, learning about our opponent and ourselves evolves naturally. The best negotiators are those who bring imagination to the table.

When we disagree but approach the situation with temperament, mutual interest and active listening, most conflicts can be resolved by the interaction of the principals involved through negotiation. We must set the stage for negotiation. Negotiation is about exchange, discovery of interests, a willingness to compromise, all to produce an action, outcome, or decision. The result must weigh both authority and responsibility typical in health care systems where authority recognizes who decides, but responsibility names who is accountable for results. Negotiation is colored by the dynamics of recognition and status and one's relative position in the traditional hierarchy of relationships within the medical delivery system.

Techniques to improve negotiation and communication skills always begin with active listening without interruption or judgement. Active listening means one assimilates and synthesizes everything one is hearing, not what they wish to hear. Your responses will range from agreement to acknowledgment and often include self-reflection. One's position statement often begins with a summary disclosure of the opponents view, such as: "Let me be certain that I understand what you are saying..." Even when you disagree vehemently with the other side, instead of attacking and creating a defensive opponent, simply acknowledging their position with a statement like: "You seem very concerned about (whatever the issue is)..." means you neither agreed with their statement nor acknowledged it as legitimate, but you listened and confirmed you heard them. Your opponent is telling you their desires. If you respond to underlying interests, this sends a potent signal that you are receptive and empathetic to what they value.

Acknowledging everyone's underlying interests opens a new, implicit question: is it possible to find a resolution that satisfies the interests of everyone involved? You must validate your opponent's view. This is a respectful and important exchange for health care professionals. Validation and its rewards emanate from an appreciative comment, acknowledgment of vital information, and the capitulation of decision-making authority. For example, a nurse practitioner might notify a supervising physician of certain facts, intent on communicating what he believes is an important piece of information about a patient. The implicit negotiation in the conversation subconsciously reasons that: 'I expect you to recognize my information as significant and therefore I am a valuable and contributing member of this team.' Therefore invalidation and dismissive remarks by the provider negating a piece of information, or excluding this colleague's participation based on prejudice, hierarchical standing, or interpersonal relations, leads to resentment, alienation, and the desire for retribution. This is costly and hurts the interdependent negotiations and work of health care, resulting in unresponsive personnel with emotional distrust between patient advocates.

Enter every negotiation with the intention of learning. Be inquisitive and explore the opposite position to the argument.

Successful negotiators have the capacity to consider all angles of a dispute, comprehend complex problems and develop integrative solutions that respect the various stakeholders' autonomy. Use Fisher and Ury's technique of reframing to 'separate the problem from the person.' This will unburden the parties and relieve everyone from guilt or shame because of their position. Respond by saying, 'I understand your position on this matter is .... which I may disagree with however we are both highly educated, and I respect your insight and commitment to resolve this issue.' This tactic transforms your opponent and encourages them to both listen to your viewpoint and seek common ground solutions with you. Especially when you worked with people successfully in the past, reference that collaborative effort and discuss the prior methods used to collectively resolve issues with your opponent. This method is called "appreciative inquiry" and with this technique, the other party will reassess and adjust their perceptions and position on the current challenge.

Name the problem or focused list of problems and give them a life of their own. Divorce the issue from your opponent, so you detach the other party from their committed position. By crystalizing and sterilizing the problem as a perspective unique unto itself that generated disagreement, the opponents often abandon their passion and emotion, recognizing alternative options for solutions solved by a collaborative relationship. Understand we all have different values placed on issues comprising the conflict. Your interpretation of merit and significance is likely different from your colleague. The practice of assigning value is difficult in health care. Remember, if someone's relative worth in the conflict is diminished, that offense can fuel bitter outrage, indignation and a deep-seated desire for revenge. Immediately alter the perception of the argument by disrupting antagonism between parties. Interrupt the narrative with something unexpected like a brief antidote, a potential new offer for consideration, or follow Steve Jobs' technique and move away from the closed-door exam room and talk about the issues on a rigorous stroll around the hospital. These methods will dissolve hostile atmosphere, dislodge cognitive blocks and offer new perspective on potential solutions.

Define a problem first before jumping to any solutions. Typically, negotiating parties are quick to suggest options, and then advocate for their position without all the facts. Since the opposing party responds in the same manner, debating the relative merits of one solution over the other, warring opponents often argue immaterial positions. It is imperative that all stakeholder's establish a consensus definition of the actual problem and disregard irrelevant misperceptions of the issues. Only then, establish the goals of this negotiation. Every stakeholder affected by the issue and subsequent agreement must weigh in during the early stages of discussion.

Encourage parties who are dedicated to early solutions to simply write them down for future discussion. Make it clear that the structure of the negotiation first identifies the interested parties, then defines the parameters of the actual problem(s) and only then, methodically discussed interests, goals and requirements of each party openly and without interruption or criticism. Finally, the forum considers suggested options and solutions, attempting to conform these to the needs and requirements of each party. Individuals at this stage of conversation are less likely to demand their self-serving positional interests above the common resolutions for the entire group. Reasonable people in a negotiation will consider the best solution as an equitable fit for all parties involved, seeking to maintain civility in the relationship.

By openly discussing diverse interests and goals, you establish trust, particularly when you utilize active listening and demonstrate understanding of your opponent's needs and interests. Acknowledge the importance of their concerns, offering individualized respect. Your opponent will treat you honorably in the negotiation. Trusting that the opponent is not 'out to conquer and destroy you' ensures a productive and enjoyable relationship between parties. All parties recognize the fragility of mutual trust and likely seek a less stressful relationship, further ensuring that agreements will be honored.

Given our social connectivity, your new compatriot may function as both a resource, ambassador, or even a defender in future interactions with associates, patients and administrators. These trusting relationships establish the social army to call upon when liabilities or hostilities are directed at the provider in future conflicts. In general, every negotiation creates a potential long-term collaborative co-strategist.

When your needs, interests and goals are disproportionately established, recognizing that concessions by your opponent favor your position, always look for opportunities to find face-saving solutions for your colleague. An individual suffering defeat and publicly derailed from their demanding claims, especially when their position was toxic, needs to save face and maintain self-dignity at the conclusion of the conflict negotiation. Their peers are watching. Establish a pathway for your opponent's graceful retreat. Include them as key players executing the ultimate solution. Typically, the most combative and loudest opponent transforms into a true believer if they are given power to participate in the final resolution. Candidate Barack Obama artfully defused mounting hostility with candidate Hilary Clinton when President Obama dismissed their contentious bilateral assaults and made her Secretary of State. A brilliant maneuver that healed the democratic party for several years.

Ultimately, doing a little pre-negotiation research provides insight into what motivates the opponent stakeholders. Prior to listing your demands, encourage them to discuss options that satisfy their needs and interests. If you know what would incentivize your opponent to move toward a consensus option, save these solutions in your intellectual war chest and meter them out as concessions favoring your adversary, only if your opponent will reciprocate. Especially when the offer is of little consequence to you, these moves on the negotiation 'chess board' endear you to the process and ensure parity and equity when you request something that is of great interest to you. With every 'victory' your opponent 'wins', acknowledge their excitement and enthusiasm to secure an agreement.

Remember that even negotiations for material worth, such as money, clinic space, and call schedules could be simple. Often, these negotiations are clouded and convoluted because of history, with reputation, professional respect, and recognition more important than the actual issues defining the negotiation. Complicating current negotiations and explaining opponents' recalcitrant positions often include past grievances of inequities and resentment about a past humiliation. These factors consciously or unconsciously drive what appears to be unreasonable demands by a party. Ask up front, before the negotiations, for your opponents to identify these issues and discuss them independent of the current negotiation. Respect their perspective even if you disagree. Do not defend past action, it has no relevance. Instead, re-align their perspective by introducing equity and value into a solution that considers the needs of all parties and reframe the current negotiation as a stepping stone to a more productive and respectful relationship.

Your objective in negotiation is to modify positional demands and morph them into interest-based cooperation, exploring collaborative opportunities to discover a joint vision. By problem solving together, stakeholders identify and acknowledge disparate interests and usually brainstorm mutually acceptable options to settle a dispute and rectify a threatened relationship. Interest-based negotiators associate as collaborators, not competitors, and allow overlapping objectives to define the peace process. Establishing interdependence amongst stakeholders ensures all parties advance in their goals. Building trust and communicating honestly and openly secures the lasting rapport with confidence and collegiality.

Collaborative strategies often "increase the size of the pie" when dealing with fixed resources, providing greater and unique opportunities previously unavailable and unknown to the negotiating stakeholders. Since most health care disagreements default to distributional (fixed pie perspective) bargaining, parties "name and claim" the limited resources as their own, regardless of their opponent's needs. A collaborative interest-based negotiation dismisses this approach outright and queries how the stakeholders can work together to ensure the fixed assets are utilized to meet everyone's needs.

Be reflective in your interests and needs. Rarely are we purely altruistic in our own intent. Attribution errors are common when we passionately advocate our righteous position, dismissing the influence of emotion and past negative perception of our opponents. Truthfully, our motivations are imbued with sentiment of discontent, anger, and even retribution when facing an opponent, particularly when we find ourselves opposite to persons of authority whose past decisions disfavored our objectives. In addition, we are easily drawn into the muck of hostile debate, completely discounting the original objective amidst escalating arguments laced with colorful metaphors. Breaking that cycle and disconnecting our visceral response by engaging our pre-frontal rational cortex can be exceedingly difficult when fighting with unreasonable people.

Amidst the battle, learn by practice, to refocus your attention for a split second on an alternative narrative devoid of combative language. With each response, when the heat rises before a retort, break the conversation with an incident or situation known to both parties, such as 'you know the emergency room if getting busier every day.' The heated exchange is fractured, and your opponent is temporarily confused by the tangential thought. Immediately interject, 'we are both arguing passionately for our position and we are moving away from a joint solution. Let's take a minute here and re-group. Our time is better spent than just arguing.' By verbalizing the emotions and then refocusing on collaboration, tempers will quell. Respect should return to the conversation and solutions will slowly emerge. The best statement reframing the purpose of any negotiation is: 'I know we both want to improve healthcare and safety for our patients, so let's concentrate on ...'

Academic recommendations centered around opponents who are positional and demand in an obstinate way, recommend 'negotiation jujitsu,' designed to diffuse both tension and anger in the conflict. This requires you to maintain control of your amygdala and therefore your emotional retorts. By listening and then acknowledging the facts or premise of your opponent's argument, you effectively demonstrate respect for their needs and legitimize your adversary's concerns. Naming them separates the opponent from the original problem, reframing their position and establishing the issues as separate entities.

As discussed, this technique does not validate nor assert that you agree with your opponent's positions, only that you believe they are valid 'for your opponent'. Expressions of empathy, the ability to understand and share the feelings of another, is an excellent tool to mitigate malevolence when your adversary is escalating their positional demands in the dispute.

As an example: Nurse, Charge Nurse and Doctor discussing too frequent phone calls and delays in responding by the provider. Nurse: "When I believe there are vital sign changes that must be addressed, I will always follow protocols and call the doctor. It is unacceptable that it takes 20 minutes to get a return call!" Doctor: "I'm sick and tired of getting called every time there are slight changes in the vitals that require no treatment. A good nurse should know that we won't be changing any medications based upon these fluctuations!" Charge nurse (mediator role) attempting to diffuse the anxiety and hostility coming from both opponents: "It is obvious you both care deeply about your roles in caring for this patient, as neither of you can provide complete care without the other. Please correct me if I am wrong, I heard you both say that information necessary to establish correct treatment needs to be communicated but the frequency of the communication is at issue."

The entity 'frequency' is now the dispassionate problem. Discuss this frequency and allow the parties to discuss optional solutions. Although it is tempting to dictate these solutions, it is far better for the Charge nurse to allow the nurse and doctor to discuss 'frequency' and its parameters, developing the resolution together. Upon an agreed solution, the negotiating parties have to reiterate their commitment to the solution and promise to respect the compromise. The charge nurse decompressed the argument and redirected the issue through an alternative frame. Neither the nurse or the doctor, without the Charge nurse intervention would have mastered this negotiation. Only by divorcing their initial salvo of accusations can the conversation proceed with a non-aggressive inquiry that defines the actual problem and seeks interest-based resolution.

Often in healthcare our opponent in a discussion is competitive, demanding, and looking to exert control and influence by refusing to negotiate. This is particularly true of high conflict individuals. There are two fundamental approaches with this person. First, shift the person toward interest-based negotiation by clarifying your overlapping objectives and similar desires. Attempt to weight these common goals over demands that are clearly irrational. As the empathetic master negotiator, exploring your opponent's concerns and fears, you begin to redirect the conversation beyond their apprehensions. The art of reframing keeps the problem at arm's length to avoid either party from impassioned claiming demands. As most people, when presented with the opportunity to demonstrate empathy, will do so. Second, express your interests in a manner that would generate empathy from your opponent. This tool is an excellent method to shift a positional negotiation toward a collaborative integrative approach. But avoid disappointment if these techniques do not accomplish all of your goals. When multiple attempts fail at reframing and discussing an appreciative opportunity to work together, you must be prepared to resume a dispositional negotiating strategy.

It is critical to know exactly what you need and want, negotiating with the presumptive goal that these requirements must be met to successfully conclude your argument. By focusing on these specifics, you will limit your zone of potential agreement. Be clear and open about your objectives, mirroring your opponent's claiming approach but avoid any disparage or dismissal of their position. Don't attack your opponent, it generates ill will and when they attack, reframe and dismiss the insult as their weakness, not your trait. Being drawn into an emotionally escalating exchange will blur your focus and distract from your objectives.

Prior to any negotiated exchange you must document and protect your best opportunities if the negotiation fails. This is your BATNA, or best alternative to a negotiated agreement. In other words, if the negotiation fails, what would be the best resultant outcome you could expect. Can you live with that situation by never compromising on your core objectives? Your preconference strategy session must detail your needs and interests, determined your negotiation boundaries, defined your BATNA and performed a critical insight analysis of how your opponent's negotiation will challenge your ever goal. Make an actual list of your goals and interests, then weight them as: 'Must haves or no deal'; 'would be nice'; 'icing on the cake'. Unless the other party is willing to concede and respect your essential needs, and your alternative includes an acceptable outcome without a successful negotiation, then be prepared to walk away. As you will see, during the exchange you must be ready to reassess your position dynamically. By respecting your own BATNA, and not wavering from this doctrine during the positional negotiation, you cannot "fail" or dismiss a compromised deal as a poor outcome. Also, DO NOT reveal your BATNA to anyone else during the negotiation. Never tip your hand or voice how much you're willing to concede just to resolve a combative exchange. Success is a compromised position, even if that is close to your BATNA. The only method to a successful dispute concession is to establish your negotiating boundaries while preplanning and documenting your objectives and your BATNA.

A classic example of positional bargaining with self-interest-based negotiation (naming and claiming by one or more party) is a medical malpractice case. Anyone who has attended a mediation, elective or court ordered, has witnessed the plaintiff's lawyers and the providers insurance company setting the bounds of the negotiation. They demand $800K and the insurance company offers $25K. There are three to four exchanges following much banter (where no one except the provider really cares if medical errors actually occurred). The ultimate number maybe down in the $200K range. Even in a case in which the provider has the highest probability of victory, the insurance company would rather spend a fixed amount, usually $75k- $100K and settle the case, as that amount is the cost of defending the claim. Almost all providers will witness a shift in their defense counsel during these negotiations when they imply that settling the claim is the best alternative, even when no malpractice occurred.

The insurance company's BATNA is the defense costs and the defense lawyers know that a successful settlement at this range makes the company happy and ensures him/her future work with the insurance company. The impact on the provider, such as credentialing and the national practitioner database, are irrelevant to the other members on 'your team'. This example also illustrates why the provider should determine the negotiation range and her own BATNA. Know the consequences if you choose to agree during these negotiations. This is critical and will have a permanent impact on your medical practice.

When entering formal negotiation for any aspect of your professional career, be prepared. Do all necessary research and define the issues before you enter the room. This information includes the position(s) you believe your opponent will take and why they present these demands. Consider how you will respond to opposing arguments that are dismissive of your interests before you begin the conversation. This process requires reflective practice, assessing your own desires and how you will express yourself when you meet resistance in the negotiation. Mental jujitsu prior to the actual negotiation is an excellent tool for brainstorming options and choices when your opponent parries and rejects your position. The pathway to your needs maybe circuitous and presenting this option as an alternative can only occur when your linear thinking is interrupted pre-debate.

Preconceive of your opponent's demands, establish multiple pathways that fulfill your core interests and present an active listening empathy that acknowledges their position. During negotiations, having rehearsed the scenario of compromise to succeed, allow rebuff of your initial requirements. Do not surrender to the opposition an emotional pedestal conceived to embarrass or intimidate your presentation. It is far better to resist concessions that fulfill your opponent's demands until they agree upon the alternative route to your actual goal. When presenting your position realize that you must be willing to let go of every gold ring to reach a compromised solution. Items on your list should be passionately advocated for whether they are critical or not, but when you are willing to concede a 'wish for', trading it for a successful agreement on a critical need, your goal is accomplished.

Remember, even in curb side exchanges in the clinic or hospital, practice this art of negotiation by exploring the other persons interests. Persuade them to discuss and defend their position (without creating hostility). Interestingly, most positions are not rationally vetted and conceived. Alternative options, revealed during your discussion, presented with a logical and articulate explanation, will frame the problem in a way that an optimal result is achieved by discussing your preferred course of action. Thank your colleague for their time and smile inwardly at your mastery of the art of the deal. Rarely will you ever exercise the BATNA alternative.

In summary, consider this information when presented with difficult conflicts that requires these negotiation techniques. Conflicts that began as small past issues have evolved, become malignant, and metastasized out of proportion to simple solutions. These problems become intractable. The desire to simplify the problem list is resisted by opponents whose baggage clouds their actual objectives. Causation might be very complex. In fact, protracted disputes in which party's harbor true resentment, usually fail during direct or third party mediated settlement. Try delaying the negotiations to work on fundamental trust and communication issues. Only then can the actual conflict be discussed. Case studies also demonstrate that authorities who demand and dictate a resolution between disputants rarely see commitment by the parties once they leave the negotiating table.

The solutions established as a by-product of relationship building are the only effective methods to minimize recidivism and repetition of behavior. **As** Harvard Law Professor Gabriella Blum writes, 'people in conflict should acknowledge and encourage areas in their relationship with the opponent that are acceptable and functional, even when a severe conflict threatens the current relationship.' The negotiator should look for these conditions as opportunities to communicate and cooperate. In Healthcare organizations, examples of successful collaboration between opponents are common and that relationship must be used to demonstrate the potential for current conflict resolution. Likewise, in order to mitigate abject distain between opponents, a negotiator should identify benevolent acts by parties to highlight their altruism. This tool is imperative during heated exchanges when parties are enraged and convinced that their opponent's only concern is their defeat.

Another opportunity for a negotiated solution occurs when instability shocks the organization harboring the disputing providers. Often a common enemy (like government intervention), alternative crisis, scandal or other major disruption in the status quo, allows the negotiator to offer a change in the dynamics of the relationship as a reason to return to the negotiation table. This is particularly effective in sustained conflicts when a creative negotiator can illustrate that a collaborative solution avoids a similar crisis. The third party managing a negotiation might also effectively use social recognition effectively to achieve resolution of intractable conflicts in healthcare institutions. Successful professionals that resolve disputes exemplify behavior that avoids similar crises affecting everyone in the organization. Good will and gratitude from peers and administrators is an excellent leveraging tool used to encourage integrative solutions to protracted disputes.

Chapter Five

The Art of Mediation

In this chapter, we shall review the practice of mediation and optimize the discussion for application to the healthcare environment. Mediation introduces a neutral third-party manager to assist in dispute resolution. Not uncommonly, administrative personnel in the hospital attempt this function, even without training. This is unfortunate as valid mediation requires very specific ethical and practice parameters that require education and adherence. The Mediator functionally brings stakeholders or parties in conflict together and assists them in reaching a voluntary resolution to their dispute. By participating in the narrative, with an understanding of the psychology behind dispositional claims causing most conflicts, the mediator clarifies important issues, reframes hostility and anger, and attempts to humanize each party using empathy and understanding to introduce alternative perspectives. The Mediator neutralizes imbalanced power differentials, whether this occurs due to status, rank, gender, ethnicity or group affiliations. The mediator solicits a variety of optional solutions throughout the dialogue and repackages these as opportunities to work in a collaborative and integrative partnership. When possible, the parties choose the settlement options that fits their needs.

Generally the response time to set up and execute a mediation is brief, particularly when the conflict issue interrupts business flow, commonly experienced in healthcare. Participating in mediation is voluntary and informed. Parties cannot be coerced to attend a nonjudicially ordered mediation. Mediation allows people to provide concessions during an argument without appearing weak and belittled. Mediation is safe and confidential. An administrative mediator listens closely and is sensitized to work place hostility concerns. She will rapidly escalate legal intervention to protect an abused party. Barring these issues, everything else discussed with a mediator is confidential. Even though parties sign confidentiality agreements that protect the mediator from subsequent testimony, the mediator avoids preserving documents, providing no record of the mediation if she receives a document subpoena should the mediation fail, and the dispute turn litigious. The parties cannot use information or settlement options, nor depose a mediator during subsequent civil litigation. The court system recognizes the mediator function and protects the conversations from discovery unless a criminal investigation occurs.

The mediation process is an expedient and inexpensive way to work out individual differences while considering the needs and interests of each party. Importantly, all decisions reached in mediation are created by the people who are in conflict, not imposed on them by the mediator, an administrator, or even a judicial authority. True mediation fundamentally encourages dialogue between parties, anticipating this will promote cooperation and creative opportunities to solve problems. Since people choose their solutions, and generally sign off on a contract that ratifies their commitment, recidivism or repetition of the same conflict issues is unusual. In addition, the process creates a model for resolution of future conflicts between parties, often without the guidance of the administrative mediator. Having gone through the process, aired their concerns and frustration and worked with the opposing party, people generally accept the consequences of their own decisions.

Additional advantages to mediation include separating the people from the problem and mitigating against actor-observer attribution bias. As Ury and Fisher write in their bestselling book, _Getting to Yes_, when a mediator isolates the problems from the personalities in conflict, defensive distributional demands by opponents are defused because people no longer feel like they are being attacked. Effectively isolating issues allows adverse parties to express respect and acknowledge their adversary as a person with appropriate and sincere concerns. These are critical first steps toward collaborating on acceptable compromises. An important mediation goal is defining the continued relationship between disputing parties. Mediation is an excellent way to preserve ongoing relationships.

Healthcare staff and providers must continue to work with each other cooperatively. Mediation can eliminate problems and preserve the relationship. An effective mediator will never dismiss a person's right to legal counsel. Often in distributional disputes designed as win-lose outcomes, such as medical malpractice mediations, lawyers direct most of the conversations and parties never resolve the issue on a collaborative accord. Mediations end in agreement 70% to 80% of the time. The flexibility of the mediation process allows multiple parties and a variety of issues to be addressed simultaneously.

Mediation is often asynchronous using the technology of the day. Computer video conferencing, phone calls and email exchanges separated in time and space, best known as on-line dispute resolution (ODR), provides even more convenience for opposing parties. Mediation is certainly less intimidating than facing a judge and jury and the expense and years of waiting for a court date can be averted. By definition, a mediation avoids resolution that labels winners and losers. A settlement in mediation is not an admission of fault or guilt. The results of a mediation are contractually confidential with parties agreeing to rules ratified in the pre-mediation agreements. Should one party breech the mediation contract or settlement agreement, legal remedies hold that party liable. The opposing party often wins significant damages in this court case as the judiciary preserves mediation solutions via contract law.

The procedural aspects of mediation depend on the style utilized by the third party neutral. There are consistent goals between these various styles that regulate and frame the typical exchange. The process begins with an individual intake interview with each party, followed by a group meeting where the issues in dispute are listed and discussed. Following this, confidential individual party meetings (caucus) discuss the need and interests of the participant. The mediator will only share what each party authorized the mediator to discuss with their opponent. Since the mediator does not openly share strategies, defenses or explanations by either party, mediation is a terrible format where a litigious party participates only to 'discover' information they plan to use at trial. Once positions and issues are defined, either in caucus or in group, opponents follow the mediator's guidance and begin exploring solutions. As agreed upon solutions emerge, they are explicitly defined and then ratified by signed written agreements.

A classic ADR process is:

1. First, the mediator begin with an opening statement which includes introductions and an explanation of the process, goals and rules of the mediation. The mediator encourages each side to work cooperatively toward a settlement. At this point it is absolutely critical that the mediator affirms that the parties present have the rights and authority to discuss and settle this dispute. Not uncommonly, many businesses, including healthcare disputes, send a representative to a mediation and not the necessary higher authority who can discuss and effect solutions. Should this occur, proceeding with the mediation is ill advised. It is often a time-loss mistake to proceed without key stakeholders participating in this process.

2. Next, the mediator encourages both sides to make an uninterrupted opening statement where the person describes the issues causing the dispute and how they are affected by it. The person is not interrupted but coaxed by the mediator to openly and honestly discuss the emotional, psychological and practical impact of the argument on their professional lives.

3. Once both parties have made their statements, a joint discussion follows. The mediator uses their professionalism to temper and

reframe emotions and positions to defuse hostilities and isolate the problems, diverting attacks on the individual.

4. Next, the mediator retires to separate private conference or caucuses where the mediator often discusses the strengths and weaknesses of this party's positions and references the needs and interests of the opposing party, exploring early opportunities for settlement options. The mediator must be very sensitive to the other party's perception while these meeting occur. A mediator who spends one hour with one party and then only 30 minutes with another will usually find the later party becomes untrusting of the mediator and falsely attributes the time differential to the mediator's preference of the opposing party over oneself. The trust relationship between mediator and client is critical for the mediator to remain functional. Every effort must be made to keep the confidence of opposing parties in the mediator's professionalism to insure a beneficial mediation experience. The mediator may also caucus with each side several times.

5. Traditionally the mediator brings the parties back together for a joint negotiation to define opportunities for collaboration or agreement in order to resolve some or all of the issues.

6. The mediator then requests a signed commitment to this agreement (or may suggest parties have their lawyers review the agreement) to solidify the deal.

    Many agreement summaries become legally binding contracts. If only partial or no agreement occurs, the mediator will advise on alternative opportunities to resolve the dispute, including meeting again to continue the conversation, referral to arbitration, or finally taking the dispute to a judge in the public court system.

7. The mediator will often check back with the parties after a reasonable time to determine if the resolved issues are honored or if other issues have arisen, offering future opportunities to collaborate again on solutions.

Mediation as a practice does not rely on common law to define the negotiation. In contrast, the courts make judgments based upon case law, and rules limit evidence admissibility or what facts will be accepted when adjudicating the outcome. This can be frustrating in medically related cases but can also prevent extraneous and irrelevant information from being admitted into evidence (see cons of arbitration below). Court is often exasperating as the most important issues in a dispute, including mitigating factors, may be excluded from the testimony. Mediation allows all of these issues to be discussed. In healthcare disputes, history and tangential issues play frequent and critical influences on the current dispute and mediation allows these issues to be openly discussed.

The mediation process is utilized routinely in business, such as collective bargaining between labor unions and management. The models discussed in this manual are excellent for workplace disputes between colleagues and competitors, co-workers, and applicable to resolve personnel issues common in the hierarchical and authoritative chain of command present in hospital systems. Mediation is not limited to provider-patient or provider- staff disputes. The business of medicine, including partnership disputes, ethical decisions, and medical staff office administrative conflicts all benefit from dispute management that avoids expensive litigation. Mediation is excellent for contract disagreements, insurance claim disputes, and network provider conflicts.

As most providers realize, as a critical service-need industry, non-partner providers or entire unaffiliated hospital systems cannot participate in collective bargaining for reimbursement. This is federally prohibited as price fixing. However, policies affecting the providers within the hospital, clinics, medical staff organizations, or negotiations with insurance companies for access to patient populations are all examples of opportunities where the mediation process is extremely effective. In healthcare, process disputes and personal arguments between individuals do not necessarily involve a legal claim, but the relationships must be attended to or else a toxic work environment will result.

With this back ground, a healthcare alternative dispute resolution (ADR) advocate is an individual, regardless of their clinical expertise or medical training, who specializes in conflict recognition, definition and negotiation toward solutions. A healthcare-ADR investigates salient issues and underlying interests, understanding the nuances of relationships, authority and hierarchy. The specialist masters facilitating conciliation and intercession to resolve adversarial disputes between parties in the healthcare organization. A neutral third party employs different styles of mediation, from transformative to evaluative, narrative to interest-based, assisting those at the negotiating table to identify legitimate interests among the stakeholders; to reframe the understanding of disparate viewpoints; to trigger imaginative solutions; and to clarify the achievements and concessions offered in exchange for a mutually beneficial outcome. As the parties develop trust in the mediator's methodology, confidentiality and neutrality, they progressively reveal their underlying concerns allowing the mediator to focus on acceptable solutions. Establishing an options list and managing conversations woven into consensus is key to encouraging the parties toward a settlement. Invariably, by the time a mediator is consulted to assist in this process, the conflict has become hostile and polarized. The mediator's success stems from the fresh nonemotional perspective on the dispute and the parties involved. The mediator utilizes inquisitive and provocative questions to examine the parties' differences, and then frames effective prospects to consider, attempting to reveal settlement decisions. The mediator moves each party away from their diverging convictions and avoids the trap of advocating one position over the other, analogous to deciding who is right or wrong, but instead monopolizes upon underlying similar desires by creating transformative opportunities to resolve the conflict.

Transformative mediation methodology assumes that the fundamental relationship between disputing parties holds a relevant history and value to the opponents, so one superordinate goal of mediation is preservation of the relationship. A guiding principal employing this method, usually requiring the third-party intermediary, is improvement in the underlying party relationships by primarily exposing and dispelling bias, attribution errors, and unresolved issues that tainted the association and contributed to the current conflict. The transformative approach focuses on empowerment and mutual recognition of the worth intrinsic to the individual, rather than immediately pursuing resolution of the dispute problems. According to Bush and Folger, 'empowerment means that the parties define their own issues and seek solutions on their own.' Empowerment is not socialism and does not demand power-balancing or redistribution, but rather, 'increasing the skills of both sides to make better decisions for themselves' and for the 'restoration to individuals of a sense of their own value and strength and their own capacity to handle life's problems.' Transformative mediators maintain that power and responsibility are key issues in any conflict, and addressing these interpersonal issues supersede an opponents need for settlement or compromise. Transformative mediation encourages a mature empathetic social and cultural affiliation between individuals, building identity- based trusting relationships where parties minimize gain and relinquish primary concerns for their own welfare. The mediator heavily emphasizes mutually beneficial solutions during discourse, enabling opponents to address their current and future problem management with enlightened insight and recognition of the value of a healthy relationship with their opponent. The transformative rapport-focused experience presumes that an enhanced relationship with positive intent toward one's opponent will foster tolerance and acceptance of the opponents values and interests. An evolved rich and supportive partnership views future negotiation through a prism of collaboration for mutual gain. The cornerstone of the transformed resolution is the identification-based trust between adversaries. Matured trust between parties is further enhanced by strong emotional bonds developing from shared recognition of similar goals and values.

Narrative Mediation style differs fundamentally from transformative mediation, and critically from evaluative mediation, as its premise is altering the relational and emotional negative attribution one party has toward the other. The narrative model does not focus on problem-oriented results or settlement. These are secondary benefits resulting from the parties reformed storyline in the future relationship. The narrative mediator works through revelation and perceptions between parties using dialogue, shepherding opponents through discovery of critical interests, experiences, and preconceived bias. Narrative mediation is grounded in the theory of social constructionism, which proposes that people are the 'products of social processes' and that 'much of what we know is hardwired into our psyches by the social and cultural world around us. (Fisher)' Opponents are influenced and manipulated by their conversations, creating opposing story-lines. People interpret experiences with different truths and facts and when these diverge, individuals become adversaries. Winslade and Monk characterize narrative mediation with a unique view of conflict: 'there is no single definable reality, but a great diversity in the ways we make meanings in our lives.' Thus, narrative mediation considers disputes a manifestation of both opponents bias, who misinterpret the truth and facts about any situation as it relates to their opponent. 'The eye of the beholder is as unique as our thumbprint' and as such, conflict is this model is the inevitable byproduct of diversity of perspective rather than a narcissistic expression of personal desires. In narrative mediation, the mediator's job is to alter the opponents' perspective by gaining insight into the dispute and discovering symbiotic story lines that will isolate a dispute from the long-term relationship. The model assumes that the relationship is both positive and mutually beneficial to parties in conflict and was healthy before the dispute occurred. In summary, narrative mediation does not search for one true story, but welcomes competing story-lines and alternative story conclusions, by deconstructing the current conflict and re-framing the perspective of both opponents for an integrative conflict understanding and possible conclusion.

The narrative approach is also an excellent default strategy when a healthcare professional detects a conflict situation developing in their professional environment. Instead of an authoritarian and dispositional approach that controls the conflict by exerting 'superior knowledge and experience', the provider reframes the conversation as both an academic and personal exercise utilizing the following approach:

1. First, acknowledge the conflict, immediately informing the other party that the dispute may subvert your common goals, such as a 'superior medical practice that we accomplish together.' An

excellent icebreaker to this conversation is recognizing the opponents contribution to quality patient care and safety.

2. Second, discuss the exact dispute from your perspective and seek confirmation of a mutual understanding of the issues from the other party, focusing subsequent conversation on the actual issues instead of extraneous chatter. If prior agreements influence the current dispute, review the essence of those contracts.

3. Next, we explain, support, and openly discuss our perspectives on the issues and offer active and attentive listening to the opponents views on the situation. This requires patience and empathy, attempting to view the story from the adversaries perspective. We must be inquisitive and not condescending, arrogant or superior. DO NOT interrupt or interject opinion and solutions while someone is expressing themselves. Eye contact and recognition. If you are unsure of a point they are conveying, ask for the opportunity to reiterate what they are saying. Utilize the re-framing technique to clarify the point, attempting to deescalate any emotional baggage that is polarizing your colleague.

4. Then encourage your opponent, without appearing as a hostile challenger, to discuss why their opinion is valid and superior to

yours. Is it an opinion or do facts support their premise? Clarify all opinions from both sides in the simplest way possible and then search for synchronous views on aspects of the dispute. This provides a common ground perspective resulting in rapid agreements between parties. All agreements generate good-will and allows isolation and simplification of remaining issues that require actual negotiation.

5. Next, capitalize on the good-will process by acknowledging these solutions as evidence of successful collaboration between prior adversaries in this negotiation. Reiterate the themes of appreciative inquiry, revealing this collaboration as a discovery of common interests, and stressing that parties now hold the template of process and conversation to address remaining disputed topics. Each issue is then discussed briefly, searching for quick compromise when this is available. As the list of disputed issues diminishes, the collaboration evolves and strengthens. Often with few remaining tough ideas to discuss, parties are often mutually empathetic, abandoning dispositional claims; disavowing both bias and attribution errors concerning their colleagues. They truly desire a healthy and acceptable outcome for their opponent. Hopefully final issues are resolved, and respectful consideration creates a collaborative alliance fortifying and expanding ones professional social associations.

6. Since narrative mediation envisions a new story line of mutual working collaboration, participants ensure open and honest methods of communication address concerns in future interaction. This successful conflict resolution benchmarks a method used appreciatively, guiding parties to overcome obstacles and develop solutions as coalition members and not adversaries.

When working with a patient's large families who are variably present during medical treatment, the narrative model is quite effective. Create a storyline going forward working together with a family through a collaborative and mutually respectful model. Following group discussion, require the family to elect a single spokesperson that you and your surrogates can talk with for five minutes daily. Entrust that person to coordinate with your office to disperse all information about progress, expectations, complications and generate specific questions for discussion. Approaching these conversations and stressing the importance that both patient and family are informed and participating in all aspects of care, creates an integrated team working in concert for a common goal. The disease is the conflict, and your collaborative team members entwined with identity-based trust, develops a storyline together that respects the provider's decisions even when adverse outcomes occur.

The Interest based model deconstructs the mediation process into simple steps, concentrating on solutions and deemphasizes the need to transform relationships or develop an alternative storyline. Fundamental perceptions of adversaries are less important. In this model, each party states his or her interests, or what the party anticipates is their gain by negotiation. The mediator follows with a discussion of overall interests where the parties, having heard all desires, list what they view as points of agreement among these interests. Next, these enlightened interests allow opponents to work together and craft new ideas and solutions previously undiscovered or not contemplated. Then, by aligning interests, and negotiating opportunities, the parties might finalize agreed upon options. The model in detail steps looks as follows:

1. The mediator assembles key stakeholders into a single group.

2. Each principal articulates their "self-interests" informing all others by claiming their desires. The mediator queries in detail, what must the principal achieve in this exchange.

3. Overlapping interests emerge and these expanded interests demonstrate opportunities for agreement. Common goals often dwarf areas of contention.

4. The mediator then encourages collaboration to achieve resolution to the remaining disagreements with creative problem solving.

5. As agreements are articulated, they are defined as 'aligned interests' as the mediator continually reframes ongoing discussion through the optics of achieved solutions. Should difficult disagreements cause the mediation to drag on, the mediation is stopped, ratifying solutions by decree or contract.

6. Future negotiations are scheduled, concentrating only on the oppositional positions of principled parties, but reminding them of the successful points of agreement so far.

Interest-based mediation works well within healthcare organizations. Common goals between disputing parties include high quality service, excellent outcomes, patient satisfaction, and adequate reimbursement while assuring medical care remains affordable. Using an interest-based approach, the mediator ensures a structured reproducible process with inclusion of all key decision-making stakeholders required to maximize opportunities for dispute resolution. The structured process minimizes both ego battles and tangential scuffles by keeping all parties focused on productively resolving the central issues. Identification and subsequent inclusion of all relevant principals is essential since people only honor solutions they help create and ratify. Without a third party neutral, one party often attempts to impose ideas and values upon their opponent and naturally they encounter defensive resistance.

A mediator dedicates pre-conference time and effort to individual conversations, clarifying problem description to avert frustration at conference when searching for common ground solutions. The mediator avoids the 'evaluative' role, disclosing her opinion on the significance of each claim or solution. Often however opponents request this commitment by the mediator when the focus of mediation is distributive, fighting over liability and monetary issues. Interest-based mediators utilize evaluative techniques when requested but attempt to redirect parties away from position-based negotiation. Instead of exclusively deliberating over money transfer required to settle a case, an interest-based negotiation in healthcare identifies the plaintiffs' noneconomic needs. These include information, an adequate apology when appropriate, a commitment that errors or omissions by providers are identified and systematically addressed, protecting future patients from similar complications. Interest-based mediation is particularly appropriate in medical malpractice cases where plaintiff patients are naïve to the complexities and uncertainties implicit in medical care. A distributive litigation rarely answers questions concerning adverse consequences of treatment and absolutely fails to separate a provider from attribution accusations of bad faith and negligence.

Interest- focused mediators invite active participation of plaintiffs and providers into joint communication sessions and utilizing both group and caucus conversation, allow patient plaintiffs to express their emotions. In addition, the mediator encourages the provider to share their emotional and psychological perspectives to ensure the patient that their provider is sincere and desires a best medical outcome. The interest-based mediator will not predict the outcome of litigation and will respect parties' decision not to settle. Lastly, in distributive claims such as medical malpractice cases, an interest-based negotiator utilizing aspects of evaluative mediation, only shares his guarded opinion about the settlement value late in the mediation. Attorneys using medically trained mediators favor the experience. Lieberman quotes several advocates: 'The mediators went to great lengths to understand claims, explain issues, and find solutions. [They] made clients comfortable with the process. The approach was [more] than beating the person over the head. [They] made useful progress in moving the case along even without settlement.' 'Most mediators are more aggressive, offering only money suggestions'.

Interest- based mediators discovered that a percentage of both defense and plaintiff lawyers wanted the mediator to opine on the money value in a case, therefore utilize evaluative input. As Dauer points out, attorneys who prefer mediators who predict trial outcomes and assign a monetary value to the case, also want the mediator to browbeat parties into settlement. These lawyers are unfamiliar with classic mediation ethics and practices, equating the process with the familiar litigation setting of a judicially conducted settlement conference. They are used to clients not participating in settlement conferences ensuring that only legal and monetary issues remain the topics of discussion. In these conferences the judge is the ultimate and forceful decision maker. As Riskin and Welch point out, 'one of the great promises of mediation ... [is] its potential for loosening the pinched perspective that typically dominates litigation practices and settlement discussions.'

An example of interest-based mediation is the *Exchange Strategy* for managing conflicts in healthcare. The Exchange program is a mediation which facilitates communication between disputing parties. A trained nurse manager, neutral provider, or a conflict professional assuming the mediator role, identifies the key parties and initiates the dialogue in a structured manner. Like all other models, the Exchange process encourages people to participate in problem solving in ways that preserve their dignity and give them input into decisions that affect their lives. The Exchange is not about discipline; it is about solving a problem. As in other models, the key components are an exchange of information or "facts" from each party's perspective and then assistance in understanding the issues and viewpoint of the opponent. These perspectives are reframed to underscore the impact and negative affects the conflict has on each party. The focus is on understanding and empathy with the opponent' position, avoiding quick resolutions or tacit agreements. The mediator initiates conversation about mutual expectations and desired outcomes, exchanging ideas on opportunities to manage and resolve the conflict. As parties are participating and influencing the process, they comply with agreements or settlements much more often than solutions dictated from administrative authorities.

The common workplace disputes a healthcare mediator manages includes: respectful treatment between staff; acceptance of different work styles; fairness in work division; recognition for contributions made by individuals; safety concerns in the work environment; behaviors viewed as compromising to patient safety; work place satisfaction; trust between staff members; and teamwork instead of individualism. Persons interviewed in medical field disputes often claim their effectiveness, concentration and contentment with the healthcare practice is threatened by the conflict. Despite an effective mediation, using the exchange method or any mediation style, mediators are not attempting to influence parties to easily transform into friends, but a manager mediator should insist that coworkers maintain a respectful and civil professional working relationship.

The Exchange interest-based mediation approach:

1. Data-gathering stage for the mediator facilitating the process. This is a private, one-on-one meeting with each party in the dispute. The mediator provides a safe nonjudgmental atmosphere exploring the parties perceptions of the situation, including preparing the opponents to discuss the impact of this dispute on each individual. **True interests are revealed by developing the "why" around this dispute, discussing motivations, expectations, fears, hopes, or concerns that led to the actions involved in the situation. It is important to allow each party to vent.**

2. Next a private-planning opportunity for the mediator to develop her agenda. The facilitator reflects on the issues and sentiment expressed and devises an agenda using conflict-resolution strategies that encompass both the upcoming joint conversation and the problem-solving process. Through inquiry, the mediator might understand how this conflict escalated beyond a simple disagreement, exposing latent and hidden issues between opponents that could emerge and impact the current negotiation. Mediators address these issues before the group session as any resolution that avoids or dismisses these issues will fail as parties succumb to future

disputes, resulting in frustration, blaming and deeper animosity.

3. The parties then participate in group dialogue, reflecting on the significance of this conflict in their lives. In medicine this meeting should never be about assessment of someone's clinical skills, but instead, foster a stimulating conversation about work styles and relationships. This provides the participants an opportunity to address salient issues in a holistic way, not just superficially by declaring a truce. The mediator facilitates respectful communication required of all parties. **In the exchange process, the manager or authority person** has a clear responsibility to reinforce workplace policies and behavior. These include teamwork and quality patient care. The mediator must stress in caucus and in group session that the meeting is not a disciplinary session but conversely, an opportunity to improve the working relationship between the parties.

4. The mediator encourages participants to express grievance in a positive verbal exchange using reframing when discussing both emotional and factual issues. As each issue is revealed, the mediator defines the problem and ensures all parties understand the issues identically. The facilitation becomes

an honest discussion that is uninhibited and uninterrupted. As individuals reveal needs and interests, a respectful counterpart assists in transforming the relationship and addressing the problems. As issues are discussed, opportunities for settlement emerge.

5. Lastly, the problem resolution phase is quite different than the earlier adversarial posturing. Colleagues begin to explore options and collaborate on practical and lasting resolution for their dispute. All mediators recognize that saving face and avoiding embarrassment or humiliation during discussion is critical. These individuals must reach a solution that does not devalue the participant, particularly when these parties must continue a supportive integrated working relationship.

The Evaluative mediation model. Leonard Riskin, a well-known attorney and dispute academician, describes the evaluative mediation model, separating it distinctly from interest-based collaborative techniques or 'facilitative mediation.' The key features noted during an evaluative session include: the mediator assesses the strengths and weaknesses of each side's arguments; develops and proposes key elements for dispute settlement; predicts how the court might decide the case; urges and pushes parties to accept a compromised settlement; and educates or lectures each party about the issues the mediator deems important. In evaluative mediations, the mediator focuses on the party's legal rights, referencing case law, while providing problem oriented, solutions-based advocacy designed to persuade the parties toward settlement, not collaboration. The mediator structures the process and directly influences the outcome by providing their perspective on claims and defenses. Riskin himself questioned if his evaluative mediation methods were defined as mediation at all. In rebuttal, Stulberg wrote 'only the mediator who adopts a suitably ... facilitative orientation is in a position to ground an approach to problem solving.' He essentially implied that facilitative mediation, as with any mediation, requires mediator to influence with evaluative techniques. Stulberg further maintained that the model of mediation was a mute argument, as proper analysis demonstrates that evaluative and facilitative methodology is identical. The evaluative mediator structures the exchange enthusiastically, instituting a sequence of events, encouraging negotiation, collecting alleged facts, evidence and arguments, and providing information. The mediator further opines and advises, altering tone, timing and content based upon the emotional and cognitive positional demands from either party.

An example of the evaluative method and mediator influence is witnesses in court ordered pre-trial mediation in a medical malpractice litigation. In these cases, both parties have "substantive opinions" introduced from "dueling experts." As an evaluative engagement, the mediator functionally facilitates discourse between opponents while providing compelling advice to both parties based upon the theme of the dispute. In reality, it is rare that the parties involved in med-mal litigation have any desire to maintain a relationship after claims are made and defenses rendered. Thus, an evaluative process with an engaged mediator focusing on acceptable settlements uses the techniques of alternative dispute resolution to avoid adjudicative litigation, limiting resolution to distributive conclusions. As Craig Pollock points out 'one well known mediator, the late David Shapiro, was known to argue that the major difficulty he encountered with party representatives was their tendency to "fall in love with their own case" and the job of the evaluative mediator was to break up the love affair.' As a student of conflict management, the healthcare provider will challenge the concept that a court ordered pretrial med-mal case mediation even approaches the definition of an elective process. Providers routinely complain these closed-door sessions border on coercion to settle and avoid trial. The legal system is truly foreign to healthcare practitioners.

Medical malpractice cases reach mediation by several routes. There might be state or court requirements, hospital dispute resolution protocols, or individual decisions to hire private mediators. Some states require parties in all civil litigation to attempt settlement through mediation. For example, title 5, section 44.102 of the Florida Annotated Statutes (1999) gives courts the power to order parties in all or any part of contested civil lawsuits to mediate with few exceptions. Title 6, section 6-6-20 of the Alabama Code (2000) allows mediation for all parties when the parties agree, on motion by either party, and when the court orders the dispute into mediation. The Alternative Dispute Resolution Act of 1998, codified as 28 U.S.C.A. § 651, requires each federal district court to devise and implement its own alternative dispute resolution program to encourage and promote the use of ADR. Thus, many federal district courts have mandated mediation. In addition, judges often suggest that parties try mediation, even where no formal requirement exists. Court ordered mediation typically requires parties to participate in at least an initial mediation session and then decide whether to continue with follow up sessions designed to reach an agreement.

In the author's experience, medical malpractice court ordered case mediations are leveraged opportunities designed to influence a physician to acquiesce toward a monetary settlement anytime a patient care issue results in less than optimal outcome. In practice, the defense insurance company, (with or without a provider's consent to settle the case) makes decisions based upon legal theories in the case, often ignoring the spectrum of possible care pathways the provider used when treating the plaintiff. Many, but not all insurance carriers require the provider to agree to settle the case and attempt to influence the provider to opt for settlement during mediation. There is greater weight placed on the plaintiff's experts authoritative claim that the defendant provider is guilty of medical malpractice, even when strong defenses are presented.

As a participant in such discourse, the author found that advocates concentrate more on the personality of the judiciary, and the likability of a medical expert, dismissing defenses that complication from care provided are simply one of many possible outcomes discussed prior to treatment. As an expert consultant, the author witnessed emotional and dispositional demands from prior patients claiming negligence, flamed by a malevolent legal representative, ignoring needs and interests beyond a monetary prize. The defendant providers are dumbfounded and indignant with the allegations. Lastly, every provider must realize that once they consent to settlement, they are irrelevant to the process. Providers often just wish to return to practice and escape the dark litigation circus, presuming that a weak case would settle for a small number. This is ill advised. Often a significantly greater amount, outrageous in many cases, is agreed upon by defense and plaintiff. The provider must bear the consequences on their credentialing and licensure, and even insurability, as these large settlements are posted on the national practitioners database. Once a provider agrees to settle, they have lost all power and influence in any case. An agreement to settle shifts the overall liability back on to the insurance carrier. So, if the case went to trial and the provider's claims-made policy limit was $1,000,000.00 per incident, the insurance company would be liable for this one million dollars plus all other damage awards decided by the court. Alternatively, if a provider refuses to settle a case and the scenario above is repeated, the provider is liable for all costs above the one-million-dollar award. The position is precarious, the stakes high and the impact may be disastrous for the provider's livelihood.

From a physician's perspective, mediation should provide emotional and psychological healing opportunities for all parties involved in the dispute, including the provider. Proper conflict management should include medical subject matter experts as a welcome alternative to the legal authorities that dominate the current alternative dispute resolution roles. The best-case scenario in healthcare conflicts in mediation requires both a medical and legal representative as co- mediators and third-party neutrals, evaluating the medicine and legal issues present in each dispute. Together the mediators balance the influence of case law, events and expert testimony, then discuss all issues with the parties. As a team approach, this mediator combination provides objective analysis of options for each side. The patient/plaintiff would can hear from a neutral lawyer and a healthcare mediator specialist. Defense nuances and judgements in care delivered are appropriately interpreted and conveyed as strengths for a defense verdict. In contrast the same impartial healthcare mediator will also embolden a plaintiff if the medicine practiced was indeed below acceptable standards. In this way, a true and fair consideration can be made on appropriateness of settlement which, as a value-added service, dramatically impacts the valuation of claims and monetary settlement paid by an insurance company.

As an example, when the author is consulted as the medical co-mediator, I discuss the case in depth with experts from both adversarial positions and utilize impartial and uncompensated care providers to ferret out important issues in a case, all completed before attending the formal mediation. This balanced approach is a critical service for plaintiff lawyers who proceed with great risk and professional exposure when prosecuting marginal cases inspired by overly enthusiastic paid experts.

As Love and Stulberg pointed out, co-mediation, 'while not common in commercial mediation, provides the benefits of increased expertise, insights, energy, and focus as well as the opportunity for one mediator to take risks.' An impartial mediator with medical training is invaluable to attorneys on both sides of the dispute, to the medical malpractice insurance companies, to hospital administrators who recognize the value of a medical expert wearing an ADR hat, and individual providers searching for an objective influence over their administrative struggles.

Facilitating discovery of needs and interests.

One of the most effective assets in the mediator's tool box are the inquiry question he develops to reveal the needs, interests and goals of the subjects involved in the conflict. As Kerri Quinn-Schmidt points out, by 'asking powerful questions' during the facilitation process, the mediator stimulates the parties journey of self-discovery, revelation and expression of their true agenda. Prior to a mediation, the facilitator neutral researched back ground information on the dispute and the individuals involved. The mediator is cautious that this information not create a bias in perspective that would limit her open inquisitive exploration during caucus with the participants. It is not appropriate to predispose, or judge behavior based upon limit knowledge, so the mediator must develop a mature and trusting relationship with all stakeholders, lest the process be weakened and ineffective. Questions should be designed to illicit specific and necessary information. Interests and goals are explored, discussing the conflicts impact on the personal and professional lives of opponents. These are frequently difficult conversation and the mediator utilized diversity of approach and reframing conversation throughout the inquiry. As an educator,

Professor Schmidt is a fascinating wordsmith, altering the language of inquiry to address both intent and goals behind the mediator's questions. For instance, the implicit meaning behind 'should' vs 'could'. As she points out, 'Should can be interpreted as a judgment. Could examines possibilities.' 'Questions have great power because they demand answers. So, it's important to formulate a good question. Define your purpose in asking the question by first asking yourself: why am I asking this and what do I hope to gain with this question?'

The facilitator understands the difference between open - ended versus closed - ended questions. To summarize, open-ended questions require subjects to contemplate and create an answer, encouraging conversation, opinion and positions. The questions create the opportunity for exchange and allow the participant to consider alternative ideas and theory as part of the conversation. Open-ended questions motivate subjects to clarify and explain, allowing the facilitator to appreciate the motivation and perspective of the individual. Free flowing conversation, actively received by the facilitator can quickly define personalities, identify road blocks, reveal unexpected goals and interests and weave a tapestry of possibilities when the facilitator searches for commonalties to bring opposing parties together. These techniques are very useful during all stages of an interest-based mediation. After one side makes a statement or takes a position, ask the opponent the open-ended question, 'What did you hear him/her say?' This question challenges the opponent to reframe their adversaries intent, clarifying positions and illustrates the importance of active listening.

Alternatively, asking closed ended questions expects a definitive answer, such as yes or no, without an accompanying explanation. These are important information gathering questions and used to reiterate an important point made by one opponent when the other appears disconnected or lacks understanding. For instance, the facilitator asks a close ended question to underscore the position of one of the parties, 'Did you mean...or Did you hear her say...' Although discussion may follow, the facilitator is securing an information bookmark in the conversation that will refence one sides position. The facilitator can alter the intention of a question by changing a closed ended question into an open-ended question by inserting an adverb such as 'what', 'how' or 'could'. As an example, 'Did that statement from your opponent surprise you?' vs 'Could you tell me how that statement surprised you?'

Professor Quinn-Schmidt discusses intended consequences of the question and answer process. As she illustrates 'try substituting "what" for "why." "Why" tends to put people on the defensive. "What" asks for more descriptive replies. During intense exchanges between adversaries, one party often directs an accusatory 'why' question at their opponent. "Why did you do...". The mediator is wise to defuse the intensity of a question that demands a defensive response, allowing the respondent an opportunity for a thoughtful explanation. The facilitator interrupt the exchange and reframes both the question and its intensity by asking the first party, 'If I hear you correctly, what you are asking for is an explanation regarding...' These quick deescalating techniques allow the facilitator to moderate temper and tempo during the exchange, fostering unfiltered but respectful dialogue between parties who refocus to answer the mediator's probing inquiry.

Anyone attending a deposition will identify the classic method of questioning taught in law school. These are leading questions designed to generate an affirmative or rejection of the proposition offered as part of the question. For instance, 'Isn't it true doctor that by operating on this patient's spine you put the nerves at risk of injury?' How to answer this question! The lawyer wants a "yes" and the surgeon wants to qualify a response. The facilitator must be careful with these leading questions as a party answering them will quickly become defensive. They are better used to establish process when the answers are 'yes or no.' Attempting to illustrate self-incrimination or recrimination derived from purposeful facilitator questions is an inexcusable ethical violation by the mediator. Therefore leading questions must be framed to a normative conclusion accepted as indisputable by both parties and woven into the question carefully. As an example: 'Isn't it safer to have open communication between nurses to avoid mistakes in medications administered to the patient?' The obvious "yes answer" is non-threatening, even when the parties know the foundation of their dispute is based upon violation of the normative value, resulting from miscommunication and the subsequent tension created. The facilitator establishes important and valid information acceptable to both parties utilizing these techniques.

As the facilitator elicits the stories from parties, she focuses on key points that impact the discussions relevant to the disputant. It is important to dig deeper and develop probing questions that explain someone's opinion, desires and goals. 'Tell me more about..' or 'Please explain what you meant when you said...' As participants in the process begin to open up, their real desires are expressed. They are relating facts while expressing their feelings and emphasizing points that are most significant to them. When common goals overlap between parties, the facilitator monopolizes on this fertile exchange, developing collaborative action and steers parties to develop those opportunities. In addition, clear communication dispels ambiguity as parties crystalize their issues, fostering negotiation and compromise, elevated above emotional intensity, and moving forward in synergy.

Facilitators develop their own conversational style, but like any story, when a party can tell what happened and how it affected them, the mediator will gauge key talking and pressure points and expand on those topics. In addition, the third party moves from past to present impact by shifting from 'How did that affect you?' to 'How is this affecting you?' The shift seems subtle but is deceptively important. When people assign blame, they do so by naming past actions as a manifestation of bad behavior. "They did this or that". Often many of those issues are irrelevant so a facilitator reframes to the present tense to reveal current issues. With this technique, the facilitator alters the conversation toward solutions with 'how' questions. When pain points are activated, 'how can the parties address this issue to work together in the future?' To progress to resolution, propel a conversation from the present to the near future. Project what new opportunities might exist with 'imagine' using 'what or how' questions. 'Imagine it is this time next year. How will you feel if this issue was (or wasn't) resolved?'

Here are some simple questions during the process of inquiry used by seasoned mediators: "What do you hope to accomplish today?" ;"What happened when....."; "Tell me about your relationship with..."; "Why do you think so-so acted this way?"; " Tell me about how you feel when you hear (the opponent) say that?"; "Can we go back to the problem of how to repair damage to the..?"; "Can you go further into that?"; "Would an apology help you overcome the emotions you are experiencing"; " What do you mean by...?"; "Tell me what you believe we need to accomplish today"; "How do you feel we are doing as we try to accomplish resolution."

Lastly, once disputants share their perspective and problems are reframed as opportunities, the mediator must continue to divert attacking language directed at one opponent. The mediator reiterates the benefits of collaboration and how the relationship will work in the future. In a healthcare establishment, have opponents predict resolution and describe their vision of effective interaction with the current adversary. This creates goals that warrant action by both parties. Often this step requires mutual apologies encouraged by the facilitator. A pervasive theme of mutual respect between collaborators celebrates each other's experience and opinion. The mediator completes successful discussions with a bilateral commitment to execute and adhere to agreed upon decisions. This includes the facilitator following up with scheduled phone calls, emails and as necessary, joint meetings with all stake holder parties. Never assume that a cumbia moment during mediation automatically transforms behavior. The facilitator must challenge the parties to focus on continued open communication and revisit the collaborative relationship frequently. There should be a low threshold to re assemble the group and rework through old and new problems.

A facilitator's services throughout the system design orchestrates a systematic approach to negotiation while not advocating for any position, thus avoiding undo influence or power in the negotiation. Frequently one side, especially if they have legal counsel, tries to influence the negotiation by executing an evaluative proposition on specific points in order to subtly persuade the third parties neutral intent. The mediator must quash that behavior and avoid agreeing with one party. Acknowledgment is not agreement. A mediator granted decision making authority in a dispute is no longer mediating, they are arbitrating a conflict. Therefore the mediator and facilitator should recuse himself from any decision-making authority or influence over any 'deal,' even when employing evaluative techniques requested as a subject expert in a healthcare conflict exchange. All party stakeholders are reminded of the mediator's role in negotiations to avoid confusion, bias or claims of prejudice by disaffected parties.

Interceding in a healthcare conflict situation, either as a primary stakeholders, or a third-party participant, uses dialogue and reframing to change the narrative. This involves improved communication and honest expression between parties. When people fight or take a defensive posture, our amygdala constructs barriers that interrupt free thought. The building blocks of this wall are emotion and paranoia. A principled view becomes quite myopic as one opponent refuses to believe their opponent can ever be effectively objective. The trained third-party is frequently necessary as a buffer in heated exchange. This model is ideal during disclosure of adverse outcomes to patients and their families. Disappointment, guilt and stress, along with a healthy influence of pessimism and litigation worry, often stunts a provider's ability to remain empathetic and communicative with patients and family following suboptimal outcomes. Private or employed third-parties, such as a healthcare ombudsman, effectively assist the provider in preparing for disclosure, projecting both empathy and compassion toward the patient. This requires practice and a carefully worded accounting of adverse events related to the patient and in the medical record.

As an expert consultant in neurosurgery litigation, the author repeatedly encounters stoic surgeons speaking very little to the family. When they attempt a conversation, they appear aloof, dismissive, arrogant and defensive. In addition, providers frequently perseverate and speculate in the medical records, not recognizing they jeopardize a malpractice defensive position should litigation proceed. The ombudsman or healthcare facilitator has practical tips and is an excellent sounding board for a health care professional who must compose an apology for any miscommunication or disclosure. For intense interchange, the mediator has a psycho-social perspective that offers opportunity for collaborative solutions between provider and patient/family. The mediator provides the framework for the provider to address the current care management communication, available now to the practitioner for future conflict exchange. These include tools and techniques to ease family fears resulting from misunderstanding or confusion during their medical care experience. The effective healthcare ADR consultant should be available to all providers practicing both inpatient and outpatient medicine.

Apology

When appropriate, apology comes framed in respect and acknowledgment. An empathetic apology following an adverse outcome is disclosure without admission of guilt. This communication is often mandatory, ratified in hospital medical staff bylaws. Apology statements acknowledge the families experience of frustration and disappointment, identify the unintended consequences of treatments, take responsibility for the situation without admitting a mistake, and communicate regret for unintended outcomes. These disclosures can decrease blame and anger, increase trust, and improve the provider-patient relationship. The laws of disclosure do vary by state and there should be a hospital expert identified through the risk management office that participates in this family meeting. Healthcare providers are cautious to avoid statements that name and claim medically negligent practices that deviate from regional standards of care. The apology encounter is not the time to fall on one's sword with regretful positional statements unless a protected apology is secured as a matter of law within the state where the misadventure occurred.

The apology is followed by a narrative approach, creating an alternative storyline, moving forward together, provider and patient, with trust and understanding that providers are human and practicing with the best of intentions. It is prudent for every provider to discuss the template for disclosure with the risk management office in their facility and to openly and actively pursue mediators and possibly legal counsel when managing extremely disgruntled patients or family members. The risk management department actually exists for non-punitive reasons and their primary goals is collaborate management, addressing concerns and interceding during adverse situations. Risk management personnel routinely call for early third-party intervention to quell fear, anger and distemper from unhappy patients and families.

Apologies should go both ways. When an obvious adverse outcome is not the main reason for a third-party to intervene with a disgruntled patient, the mediator must ask the parties to acknowledge the dispute and let the healthcare professional vent. This should only be done after caucus with the mediator listening to an emotionally frustrated provider's commentary on the problem. Reframing before group meetings is critical and the provider is encouraged to establish issue lists that will be digested with solutions in mind. Some common themes that instigate providers' ire and lead to miscommunication with families are: unrealistic expectations by the patient and family; too many calls that prevent the provider from caring for other patients; and a lack of respect when dealing with office staff. Both patients and their family need to hear and understand these behaviors threaten the relationship with the provider and cannot be tolerated. In these situations, it is equally important that high conflict behavior from families or patients be neutralized, removing their power position that utilizes aggressive attitudes to intimidate medical staff.

Allowing these aggressive and hostile outbursts is demeaning and demoralizing to all healthcare personnel. The energy required to deal with these personalities can be enormous and these individuals will not likely change without extensive psychotherapy. These situations are bad for the professional's piece of mind and harmony within the establishment. The mediator utilizes positional bargaining skills within the context of narrative communication, defusing an obnoxious and demanding patient by reminding them that the provider will use an authority position on healthcare matters to set the treatment and communication agenda. In addition, a toxic patient or family will not be tolerated in the practice. The patient is further reminded that outbursts and aggression jeopardize the trusting and productive relationship the provider requires to remain engaged on this patient's care management team. Over the course of my thirty-year medical practice, I have discharged several irrational patients who persist in caustic behaviors despite our best efforts.

Chapter Six

Arbitration

Arbitration is private adjudication of an adversarial dispute and utilized frequently in contracts signed by the healthcare provider. In addition, many ACO, HMO and managed care organization require patients to sign binding arbitration clauses before assuming care responsibility. Participating in contract arbitration is elective and must be selected at the beginning of a relationship before an adverse event occurs. On occasion, disputing parties already entrenched in their positions will select arbitration as a method, mid-conflict, to adjudicate their differences. Participating in an arbitration means parties are forfeiting their right to a jury trial. Although this may appear beneficial to the healthcare provider, there are significant risks associated with the arbitration process. Unlike mediation which requires parties to agree on the details of settlement, binding arbitration does not. Naïve parties frequently agree to arbitration as part of the contractual relationship they establish with an agency, yet few outside of the legal profession understand the nuances and risks of the arbitration process. Arbitration is private adjudication in which the disputing parties must hire a private judge.

The two largest American agencies acting as clearing houses and social support structures for arbitration at the time of this writing are the American Arbitration Association and JAMS, formerly known as Judicial Arbitration and Mediation Services, Inc. Arbitration formats are varied but in general, disputing parties hire a single presiding legally trained professional to preside over the case. Versions of this model generally increase the number of arbitrators, particularly in industries where a subject matter expert is appropriate, such as healthcare. These arbitrators hear the case, review evidence and render decisions. The decisions may be binding and enforceable or non-binding, in which either party may reject the findings and proceed with alternative remedies such as traditional litigation. Importantly, the parties do not decide on solutions. The parties do however have some control over who will adjudicate the case and this option, plus the private nature of the process, attracts commercial entities to the arbitration process. Because arbitration requires informed consent by contractual signature, and parties influence whom shall adjudicate their case, arbitration is attractive as an alternative method to resolve significant conflicts outside of the court system.

Arbitration does have certain advantages. In general, arbitration avoids open hostility between parties as the arbitration process encourages individuals to collaborate on the process of adjudication, recognizing that these same parties refuse to work on mediated integrative solutions. The pre-arbitration interchange can function as a peace accord, de-escalating opponents angst and animosity toward one another, allowing them to conduct the arbitration with commitment but in a professional manner. In the past arbitration was cost efficient, however this has changed as arbitrators command hirer salaries, require court reporting, and parties retain legal counsel to present their case. Additional multiparty arbitration panels increase the cost dramatically. The opponents pay for all of these services. Arbitrations usually can expedite resolution of a dispute, compressing specific legal proceedings such as motions, evidence presentation and expert witness depositions, all of which create the lengthy open court adjudicated case prosecution.

Frequently arbitrators are selected after consideration and agreement by both parties, finding the judiciary through a third-party arbitration service. Thus perceptually, this control should make arbitration fairer since, no single party in the dispute decides who the arbitrator (or arbitrators) will be. The courts consider arbitration decisions final. Although there are four conditions in which a binding arbitration can be appealed through the court system, the bar to prove maleficence of the arbitrator is so high that the decision, no matter how skewed or perverse to one party, is essentially immutable.

In many industries arbitration is superior over litigation, functionally simplifying dispute resolution by avoiding complex legal filings, prolonged discovery, multiple pretrial hearings, and subpoenas. However, a represented party with aggressive legal counsel can and will generate extensive paperwork, demand multiple hearings, require depositions, utilize subpoenas, and encumber their client with the same costs and process of a litigated case. As arbitrations have morphed into the common private mini-trial, all of the procedural steps familiar to litigators, including motions practice and legal posturing, extensive discovery, and submission of unrelated information offered to sway the arbitrator, are common legal maneuvers.

Although arbitrations have simplified the rules of evidence submissions which is divergent from the rules of evidence in court litigation, arbitration can, if agreed upon by both parties, dispense with traditional discovery such as answering interrogatories and lengthy depositions. Instead arbitrations may not rely upon testimony, but open document submission without restriction. However, if parties agree, the arbitration may require witness and expert posturing, all to influence the arbitrator toward one parties demands. This is exactly like court litigated cases. The benefit however is arbitration hearings are private and transcripts created during the process are confidential to the procedure and never part of the public record. This is valuable as the transcripts cannot become evidence for either party in some future litigation. The results, awards and judgements can be kept confidential. However, the winning party may have to return to the federal district court presiding over the arbitration location in order to convert the arbitration award into a judicial writ of execution. The writ allows the victor to enforce the judgment against his opponent. At this stage, a disaffected losing party refusing to honor the results files motions in the court to overturn the arbitration award based upon the arbitrator's prejudice, ignorance, or bias. The action is equivalent to an appeal. Statistically, federal judiciary rarely overturn an arbitrator's decision, even when the decision included mistakes in interpretation of civil law. The case, the litigation and the results of the arbitration are now part of the public record.

There are significant risks with arbitration. Costs borne by the parties escalate quickly as third-party services and legal counsel participate in the process. Arbitration varies in complexity and structure, so cost estimates are illusive numbers and unknown to parties when they agree to arbitration long before a dispute arises. Should one side disagree with an arbitration decision, the dispute is not resolved and even in binding arbitration, court action, as described above, can be pursued. This adds substantial time and costs to the process. There is a misperception that deciding upon who will be the private judiciary ensures objectivity or fairness into the arbitration proceedings. In addition, since many individuals signs contracts for services they later dispute, a binding arbitration clause, much like a court case, requires a party to participate in arbitration even for minor conflicts. Organizations and companies that require arbitration are legally prepared for the process, familiar with specific arbitrators, and utilize the arbitration system frequently, thus becoming valuable referrals to the pool of arbitrators they choose from. This absolutely creates a user bias that an unfamiliar party may be ignorant to, bound to abide by prejudicial decisions. The contractual clauses that consumers sign, including healthcare providers accepting employment with large hospital organizations, or patients entering an integrated medical delivery model, details where and how an arbitration shall proceed. The timing, cost and location often create hardship for the less powerful participant in this process.

As noted above, appealing arbitration rulings is often an insurmountable and expensive task, even when arbitrator make subjective and bias rulings. From most people, having a jury of their peers is an important right and should not be easily surrendered. This is only available through the traditional court litigated system. Arbitration eliminates that right, handing over the judge and jury role to an arbitrator. As the court rules of evidence, rules of discovery and presentation of a case do not apply in arbitration, it is exceptionally rare that a judge in the traditional court system will bother ruling on an appeal. Generally, they simply ratify what the arbitrator has decided, even if it was blatantly unfair. For this reason, should arbitration be required, all healthcare providers must demand a subject matter expert assume a co-arbitration role. This should neutralize the effect of litigator bravado as the neutral arbitrator with medical back ground balances facts over persuasive but opaque legal arguments. In the past few decades, arbitration has become a mainstay in resolving legal disputes in the healthcare system but subject matter experts as co-arbitrators are scarcely utilized.

Individuals must make an informed decision when signing contracts authorizing mandatory arbitration as the contingent dispute resolution process. In addition, knowing that formal adjudication requires arbitration, parties may be motivated to utilize mediation and try and resolve their differences. Being aware of the possible drawbacks of arbitration affords practitioners bound by contracts to participate in the process using their strategic power and authority to influence the early arbitration decisions. Providers must make careful choices, such as *who and how many* arbitrators will hear the case; if they are legally represented, how experienced is their lawyer with arbitration proceedings and selecting a competent, unbiased arbitrator. In addition, providers should discuss mediation and arbitration with their medical and business insurance carriers.

There should be provisions in those contracts that allow providers to choose their legal representatives and participate in choosing one or more mediators and arbitrators if those processes are advocated and economically supported under the insurance contract. Remember, if the arbitrator's award is unfair or illogical, the losing party must hope for the rare circumstance that an appeal is heard in federal district court and the arbitration award is over turned. The court then usually abides by the original contract, sending the case back to arbitration. The costs and time continue to weigh down the parties and the issues drag on for years.

As mentioned, many of the national arbitration groups actively market their services to large healthcare organizations and become the default agencies selected during an arbitrated dispute. One concern is always objectivity and prejudice when organizations utilize the same arbitration service and small set of arbitrators to settle their disputes. Arbitration hearings are private, and decisions are rarely publicly accessible. Thus without public disclosure or court prosecution of a claim, arbitration lacks transparency. Large organizations, particularly those prone to public recrimination for perceived wrong doing, like healthcare, favor the anonymous process and awards resultant from the arbitration adjudication. The hospital can keep the lawsuit out of the paper. Unfortunately, a process that is not transparent yet empowered with the same authority as the court systems, is prime for abuse and weakened by undue influence. Since arbitration decisions are so infrequently reviewed by the courts, the reality that larger healthcare organizations require providers and patients to default to binding arbitration is troublesome.

Although contracts requiring arbitration must be entered electively, not even legal advocated reviewing those contracts provide sufficient warning to consumers to challenge the nature of dispute settlement. One safety net when negotiating contracts is to insist upon non-binding arbitration or mechanisms within the contracts that allow either party to appeal a decision to a panel of different arbitrators. These stop gaps create clarity and objectivity to the arbitration process and decisions, even when performed through private proceedings. Much like judges, an arbitrator who knows his/her award will be critically interpreted by their own colleagues during appeal, should proceed cautiously, without bias or prejudice, providing the service that parties desire and pay for.

A provider who discovers arbitration clauses which are objectionable does have power and influence to alter the contract and protect their rights. Arbitration is not a 'bad' option as this text might represent, however knowing the risks of the process, an informed provider can utilize flexibility in contract negotiations and demand additional rights to protect future interests.

One benefit of court litigation is to limit accusations by plaintiffs to the current relevant case. In arbitration, past actions and claims do influence the arbitrator. Although the theme of ADR is generally to avoid litigation, with faster resolution and possibly lower costs, one benefit to the formal judicial process is rules of evidence submission. During litigation, plaintiff's attorneys will try and cloud the issues in front of the court through a motions practice, attempting to enter unrelated malpractice claims, credentialing issues, and professional sanctions, all as important allegations to weaken the credibility of the treating providers or hospital. The formal litigation process usually prevents most if not all of this extraneous information from disclosure at trial, avoiding undue influence on either judge or jury.

As an example, the litigation of an open medical malpractice lawsuit and strategies for the current malpractice defense. In the judicial setting, it is extremely rare for a judge to allow past claims or perceived mis-deeds by the defendant provider as evidence in a current claim. In arbitration, in which no jury is present, a single privately paid lawyer or retired judge is sitting as the sole purveyor over the dispute. The evidentiary rules for consideration of information are more flexible and defense counsel often cannot prevent claims history or other public information from prejudicing a binding arbitration process. The arbitrator often openly receives this 'evidence' and will likely be influenced by the past record of a hospital or the healthcare providers. Even when defense objects, the plaintiff parties can enter evidence as 'judicial notice,' prejudicing the arbitrator and strengthening a weak liability claim. Previous case exposure, complaints, and social media assassinations are easily introduced without restriction, damaging the providers reputation and adversely influencing an arbitrator trained only in the legal profession. In distinction, the traditional litigated court system, with its federal rules of evidence, is far more restrictive and protective, limiting a jury to the facts presented only in the current case. Arbitration is therefore a contest between the skills of articulate lawyers that weave a distorted narrative with tangential 'evidence' that should remain irrelevant to the current dispute.

The classic need for formal legal representation in court adjudication of disputes from policy, contract, and personal injury/medical malpractice cases are shifting away from exclusive judicial court environment. With the significant increase in private and binding dispute management using arbitration or its variances such as mini-trials, early neutral evaluation, case management during judicial settlement conferences, and moderated court required settlement conferences, the provider must learn all he/she can to protect themselves. When we are drawn into these adversarial disputes, these legal procedures have significant influence and pain in our professional and personal lives.

Routinely, healthcare partnerships, administration and care delivery are now governed by arbitration clauses for disgruntled parties. Healthcare professionals must understand trends in medicine that arise from adversarial positioning and educated in these alternative dispute resolution options. As more healthcare providers become co-arbitrators, the influence of the legal profession controlling the private adjudication of disputes will balance and evolve into a fair consideration of evidence and facts. Healthcare providers are considered arbitration specialists with subject matter medical expertise and should provide an objective voice while mediating or arbitrating these dispute resolution proceedings. The shift toward mediation and arbitration in healthcare dispute management requires trained professionals with both medical and legal understanding of evidence and process. As our professional roles evolve, it is imperative that practitioners assume responsibilities that allow them access to the third-party position in dispute management. The need for the medical subject matter expert to understand and weigh the relevance of the facts and expert testimony is critical.

Chapter Seven

The Healthcare Trained ADR Expert and Current Strategies in Pre-litigation

As a healthcare professional dedicates time and study toward conflict engagement techniques, they develop skills in negotiation which improves their interaction with colleagues, administration, and patients. With practice in more sophisticated ADR strategies, the provider will improve their skills when facing challenges in contract negotiation, litigation avoidance and management, investigations from peer reviews or even medical board inquiry. Conflict engagement is akin to debate preparation when the individual practitioner is one of the parties in conflict and a skilled third-party neutral is unavailable or not desired. Practitioners find themselves in competitive turmoil in the landscape of hospital systems where an innocuous inquiry may mask a challenge to one's perception of standards in care delivery. Currently the availability of medically trained skilled ADR professionals is limited so dispute management is restricted to improved communication between provider and family following adverse outcomes or formal court ordered mediation required during litigation. These merely touch the surface of the ADR opportunities for the evolving medical practitioner. A study of transformative discourse would tactically improve interaction with other professionals, especially those subordinates to the providers position in the traditional hierarchy of healthcare responsibility.

Practically speaking, conversation using empathetic inference and overtones can be practiced and mastered. Although a qualitative attribute, patient satisfaction with healthcare providers correlate highly with this skill. Marriage of intellect, technical ability and mastery in this art of discourse secures success in clinical practice, regardless of the density of competitors or administrative demands. Every provider will deliver bad news, compromised outcomes and grim options to patients and family. A practiced dialogue incorporating the skills reviewed in this manual, prepares the provider for difficult conversations and guarantees the frequent purveyor of bad news consistent discussions represented with compassion and understanding. Adopting and practicing conflict management approaches arms the provider with practical skills when responding to the disruptive and dispositional personalities of doctors, nurses and administrators who fail to embrace professional collaborative and integrative co-existence. Focusing on our own experiences through the lens of integrative transformational understanding and potential resolution is very useful. These exercises move us away from pawns inside a drama triangle, requiring a reflective understanding of interpersonal dynamics, and divorces are emotional and visceral reactions to conflict, replacing it with an academic understanding and opportunity to use the skilled facilitator structural approach.

The practitioner negotiator can avoid the extremes of dispositional and adversarial conflict arising from both divergent clinical perspectives and disgruntled patients. Currently, many programs certifying Nurse Practitioner require coursework in formal ADR education. The time invested is mandatory. Simultaneously, healthcare professionals trained in ADR provide justice to colleagues and families as an objective, empathetic but emotionally balanced voice. The value of a medical-subject matter expert co-managing adjudicated tort complaints, high conflict healthcare professional controversies, and privately litigated disputes cannot be overstated. Conflict situations requiring the practical application of the ADR discipline impact our professional lives, whether we are consenting participants or drawn into the controversy without desire or intent. The information exchange and response between care givers requires constant negotiations, fact finding and collaboration to maximize a beneficial outcome.

For the most part, despite disagreement, the issues resolve through simple discussion with reference to science. Unfortunately, the exchange may be intended as sterile communication but received as angry, demanding and dismissive. How often our brusque tone is perceived as arrogance when in reality, we are just managing and responding to the constant barrage of information. Relationships in tense environments are tenuous at best and opponents emerge from the shadows. Turbulent times trigger cascades of attribution errors. Hierarchical communities are petri dishes of discontent, rippling across a population with the speed of a paroxysmal atrial tachycardia. Disaffection breeds contempt and distrust with aggression, resulting in disregard for the population we are entrusted to care for.

Hospital and clinical culture is a rich and unique environment requiring a dedicated trained specialist in healthcare conflict resolution management. Third-party advisers and facilitators committed to educate the staff will also quickly intervene in disputes before they escalate. Traditionally, the risk management department tasks persons of various back grounds to assume the intermediary role. These professionals may not have the depth or breath of experience to handle highly educated, aggressive, high conflict personalities commonly seen in healthcare systems. Large organization such as the U.S. Armed Forces medical branches, Kaiser Permanente, and many academic institutions train ombudsman for this role. Theoretically, the ombudsmen provides functional real time investigation, collaboration and intervention between staff, providers and patients. Statistics show that their emphasis is on timely disclosure following adverse events, facilitating communication between providers, patients and family. In this limited application of ADR principals therefore, the ombudsman advocates for conflict resolution between patients and providers without assuming the patient advocacy role. This would fundamentally skew the ombudsman toward one party and impede impartiality. Unfortunately, very little time or effort is directed toward the critical need of human resource management addressing the common conflicts arising between busy and stressed healthcare professionals.

The classic job description for the medically trained ADR professional role in a healthcare system includes: implementing conflict management systems, maintaining confidentiality in all discussions, conflict coaching linking conflict resolution to quality of care and patient safety, neutrality, independence (not part of administration or HR) and informality. A robust ADR position requires flexibility as a mediator, establishing a facilitation services designed for work process improvement. An ADR specialist will not generate a formal record of the interchange between conflicting parties and is never part of a disciplinary board enacting sanctions on a healthcare provider. An example of an effective ADR systems administration plan is the dynamic adaptive model (DYADs), which utilizes and effects distributive bargaining, integrative bargaining, and interactive problem-solving models of conflict resolution, using intergroup expectancies and attitudes. This dispute management group consists of equal numbers of professionals and non-clinical persons with administration representatives. Philosophically the emphasis suggests that the common history and organizational pride and identity create synergy of purpose, heal conflict scars, and create healthy medical work environment for staff, practitioners and patients. Members of this group, using the interactive techniques to conflict situations, affect the greatest positive change in disputants, sensitive to persons of diverse cultural and clinical back grounds during successful conflict resolution.

A program developed by ADR specialists with healthcare background should focus on improving communication and supporting collegiality, identifying all opportunities when the staff are not in conflict. Training colleagues, allied healthcare personnel and clinical subordinates in conflict engagement and adverse patient outcome management, improves both safety and quality in healthcare delivery. The program then focuses upon the situations creating disputed issues which are evaluated using root cause analytics. The down line team of staff and prbviders gain insight and opportunity to recognize future potential concerns by systemic adaptation of agreed upon solutions. Conflict management is never defined by knee jerk solutions offered in a defensive or reactionary setting. The process requires an organized high-profile dispute resolution system to receive, evaluate and measure all perspectives on any issue and the subsequent impact these disruptions have upon the stakeholders. This is currently lacking in most hospitals and healthcare organizations.

Development of formal processes, easily accessed and responsive to providers and patient concerns is critical. Practitioners are acutely aware of complaints that generate peer review, quality assurance review, potential medical board inquiry, and litigation. The unspoken cost of these prolonged examinations both emotionally and professionally is enormous. Challenges to one's judgement regarding patient care following an unexpected outcome has a detrimental impact on the providers professional status and reputation. The entire experience is a painful ordeal that drags on for years of soul crushing arduous scathing battle. We cannot help but obsess on this issue. The events, decisions and all possible negative outcomes consume the providers' thoughts, interrupt their sleep, cause depression and diminish practitioners' empathy and commitment to the profession. The years of study, the need to provide economically for family, and our self-perceived identity prevents simply abandoning the profession, despite the desire to do so. Despair and sadness go untreated, subsequent errors are made and providers fear their competence will be further attacked. Hopelessness creeps in and is consuming. As a unique population, the statistics of healthcare professionals committing suicide is alarming and near completely ignored. This is the 'second victim phenomenon' where the care deliverer falls victim to the barrage of social and judicial assaults. Performing our best without intended malice is not an adequate defense and fosters no compassion or comfort from the public, courts or our colleagues.

An ADR healthcare professional is uniquely qualified to identify and intervene early in the conflicted life of her colleagues. Simply dictating institutional policy does not prevent or manage toxic disputes. The conflict manager position can positively impact the personal and professional lives of healthcare providers, avoiding the psychological poisons with structure and intervention when issues first arise. To begin, create opportunities for healthcare professionals to improve their communication techniques that mitigate adversarial interaction between staff members, patients and providers, utilizing transformative appreciative inquiry to facilitate collaborative outcomes-based best practices. Our goal is to empower the individual provider with knowledge and methods practiced in the discipline of conflict engagement. By improving the quality of our message and our strategic approach to dispute management during adversarial posturing, practitioners develop skill sets in negotiating with each other, administration, and the myriad of influential bureaucracies dictating our futures as practitioners. Combined with a clear evidence-based approach to their medical care, the enriched provider functions as a resilient advocate for their patient's wellbeing and their own practice fulfillment.

Implicit is the learning process merging the clinical experience with investigative communication, expanding our perspective on physical disease entwined with social interaction. The provider is rewarded with deep and meaningful interaction between colleagues and her patients. Practitioners climb toward Maslow's peak by providing safety to our dependents and those that depend on our skill. Instead of drowning in the quagmire of inevitable conflict, adopting the default defensive provider position, the frequent input and exercises established through an ADR office prepares practitioners to respond strategically to naïve patients demanding their entitlement to perfect health. Inevitably someone must manage the disaffected party and irritated providers. The ADR healthcare specialist is perfectly prepared for this responsibility. Through mock trial and practice, reiterated with facilitative coaching and pathway engagement, we can structure our dialogue to prevent miscommunication, deliver bad news, and navigate empathic apologies.

Case Study: the new ACO Model and role of the provider-ADR expert.

As an example, opportunities for medically skilled mediation services are presented by Roth and Fromer who write about anticipated disputes in the new accountable care organizations (ACO). They reflect upon the types of potential disputes and advocate for third party mediation to address conflicts in an expeditious and efficient manner. For back ground reference, the accountable care setting differs from traditional fee for service provider reimbursement models. Escalating costs associated with point of care third party payers created a market need for federal intervention and cost control through quality initiatives. The ACO model rewards preventative care and targeted quality care with measurable improved outcomes. The provider assumes additional responsibility and must partner with the patient, keeping them as healthy as possible.

Theoretically, overall costs will decrease by preventing complications from diseases that should be controllable through preventative management and lifestyle modification. The mantra of the ACO is that the patient must receive the right care, at the right time, and in the right setting. The ACO is therefore constructed as a group of providers willing to follow detailed evidence-based guidelines, remain educated with the most recent recommendations for care, and agree to economic bonuses or sanctions based upon the costs to care for their population of patients. Specific metrics in their population are closely monitored by outside organizations. The ACO governing board must also be a majority of practicing providers who are invested in the care of the target population but willing to accommodate their own reimbursement and practice guidelines in deference to the ACO governing body. Therefore the infrastructure of an ACO is the guidelines, benchmarks and metrics that drive quality care at lower costs. This must be done with performance measures for all providers in the ACO, who become preferred providers for the patient population.

The center for Medicare services (CMS) introduces and modifies key metrics that the commercial ACO adopts and requires of the providers working under this model. These include patient disease outcomes, quality of care process, patient satisfaction, costs to care for the population and a providers willingness to participate in the ACO, or a citizenship score. Individual providers are objectively and subjectively evaluated and receive a score card that impacts their future participation in the ACO as well as their reimbursement.

The entire ACO might be economically penalized for the poor scores obtained by a few providers. The providers risk termination from participation if their scores are not acceptable to the governing board. Medicare systems altered their payment approach based upon the Medicare access and merit-based incentive payment system in which both financial incentives and penalties are based upon quality, resource utilization, clinical practice improvement activities and advancing care information systems.

In this ACO environment, providers are expected to become integrated team members of an entire organization and relinquish individualism typical of the healthcare practitioner in Western medicine. The required complexity of communication between providers and with patients and their families are now exponentially increased. Also, the providers and their networks are held accountable for all members within the entire organization. Accountability for outcomes are now closely monitored. Anyone practicing medicine over the last twenty years understands the seismic shift impacting their practice and can appreciate the conflicts that will arise between parties interacting in this complex organizational machine.

Roth discusses several anticipated issues that would benefit from a third-party dispute resolution specialist with education in management and medicine. Issues include providers in the ACO who fail to meet the metrics requirements for disease management and are penalized or excluded from ACO participation; providers who "allow" their patients to use out of network services that are costly to the ACO which believe the provider should capture these patient encounters; severe penalties for providers who fail their citizenship participation as disgruntles patients complain about the providers personality or bedside manner despite receiving appropriate healthcare, labeling the provider as disruptive; payment disputes between providers and the ACO governing board over bonus valuation regarding work load and complexity of patients within the system; payment disputes between providers and the ACO governing board over bonus valuation that fails to quantify savings contributed by specific providers; risk assessments in the care and management of complex patients whose demands from the system and compliance with recommendations are more difficult than their healthy counterpart; and lastly disagreement over the implementation of guidelines as benchmarks qualifying care delivery decisions when patients fall outside the normative health curve or fail to respond to treatment within those guidelines, both of which damage the provider's scores. Appropriately, providers dispute the demand to take financial responsibility for these outliers.

In contrast, common disputes in managed care organizations include medical necessity conflicts, stop loss calculations, out of network treatment, prompt payment and contract case disputes. The most prevalent reason disputes arise in these contract-based relationships is over medical necessary claims following treatment. Denial of service claims for reimbursement, disputes regarding risk adjustment calculations applied to patients when determining responsibility and scoring providers relative to the loss compliance of their patient population are common.

Third-party mediation requires comprehensive understanding of medical indications for care, the impact of disease outliers on practice parameters and creative recommendations for managing these disputes is critical. Only a healthcare trained ADR specialist can fulfil this need.

The costs of litigation requiring discovery and experts in this new model are enormous. Any legal action venturing into uncharted territories creates foundational case law and the process is complex, extremely expensive and time consuming. No provider wants to be part of this process or rely on a fair adjudication of facts by parties trained in distributive resolutions where there are only winners and losers. In addition, the providers litigating the issue against their employers, HMO and ACO governing board must continue to work closely and professionally with other members engaged in this heated dispute, with difficult emotional conflict inhibiting their communication and collegiality.

A provider fighting administrative conflicts of any kind is, by most state laws, entitled to a "fair hearing process' before any administrative action can be taken against a provider. These procedures are lengthy and expensive, and providers have a right to competent representation, experts opinions, lengthy discovery, anticipated appellate action and the potential prolonged strain of litigation. These issue have a profound impact on the provider. Any adverse action is reportable to the national practitioner database. Given the option for ADR specialist intervention, many providers opt for a 'fair hearing request' utilizing mediation framework to avoid negative financial consequences of prolonged litigation and avoid disclosure of the investigation on future credentialing applications. The mediation model keeps the process confidential.

Due to the multiplicity of complex issues creating disputes in the healthcare field, the healthcare mediator will deliver all the fundamental benefits found in alternative conflict resolution doctrine. They provide control of time, expense, and distractions. The medical ADR attempts to preserve relationships, assure the continuity of patient care, allow parties to improve their communication, formulate their own acceptable solutions, and keep the process private. The healthcare mediator can assist in mitigating extensive administrative fair hearing adverse procedures. By preserving confidentiality within healthcare systems and crafting solutions to disputes not available through formal administrative litigation, such as negotiating the repercussions of any negative actions taken by a medical board or medical executive committee against a provider, the medical ADR is the provider's best option for conflict management.

Reflective Practice and Reinforcement Training.

If the healthcare practitioner is still unconvinced that conflict management skills are necessary, simply reflect upon the preparation required to professionally function and survive when administrative bodies or adverse lawyers prosecute a claim against the provider. Our social interconnection and preoccupation for scandal convince the public of sinister guilt long before one's day in court. Anyone can destroy the reputation of their opponents by initiating a hospital inquisition, medical board complaint and tort claim attack. Whether these are meritorious or not, they are expensive to defend and psychologically devastating. The disruption, anxiety and impact on the provider's mental health and clinical practice create permanent deep scars and leaves patients and colleagues with insidious doubt. Loud defenses, indignation and claims of unfair attack are irrelevant to the media. Frankly, no one cares and often no one, not even a close ally, is invested in vanquishing the assault on behalf of the provider. Even when providers prevail in court, there is little more than passing interest. The scandal sells papers, not the vindication.

Therefore, the benefit and value of a conflict management mindset is premeditation, to guard against these situations. For providers believing their reputation and time served for the community will protect them, this simplicity may be their undoing. So, from my years, deep scars and tactical successes, the author encourages learning these lifelong professional skills and strongly advocates for the healthcare trained ADR professional to be able and available at every medical institution. Avoid disputes with colleagues because of competition over who provides superior care when you disagree about treatment or intervention. Educate oneself and maintain proficiency in collaboration, openness, and disagreement resolution instead of rivalry to conquer. Practice to preserve your sanity and professional well-being.

A subject matter medical dispute manager is instrumental to facilitating and addressing the critical void in current litigation and adversarial platforms. By providing the mandated neutral balance with objective understanding of the healthcare environment, the medical ADR offers a neutral and nonbiased collaborative approach to mediation and arbitration in healthcare disputes. When the practice of medicine is overwhelmed by procedural manipulation during legal quarrels, a healthcare ADR specialist skilled in negotiation and conflict engagement will objectively neutralize the dispositional bias found in the legal professionals.

Currently lawyers alone dominant the mediator and arbitrator practices of our private justice system. A healthcare provider adds administrative and procedural balance to a preoccupied adversarial approach common to legal counsel. It is not necessary to accept an exclusive lawyer driven process that focuses on economic victory. The truth inherent in the care decisions must be understood and integrated into every mediation discussion or arbitration process. The healthcare ADR expert is a keystone of successful procedural collaboration between lawyers and should be present on all medical legal panels. A medical ADR expert balances the process and assures that any plaintiff, their lawyers and paid experts, truly understand the medicine practices and the ramifications of the care provided.

Providers are reminded that the current mediation and arbitration process is evaluative and dispositional and there is no collaboration or neutral impartial communication using traditional mediation services. We should be cautious when 92% of litigated medical malpractice cases settle before trial even when the merits of the case do not support a plaintiff verdict. Unfortunately, in this process the defendant healthcare provider, being surrounded by lawyers, are often harangued and coerced into accepting a "mediated" settlement because there is no neutral voice evaluating in caucus whether the standards of care were violated, the veracity of expert witness testimony, and truly communicating if a claim will withstand the test of judicial inspection.

Long before lawyers gain the bully pulpit, a medical ADR process administered at the clinic and hospital will address provider errors and conflict behaviors. The systems in place establishes several core needs, expressed as institutional values, codified by the medical and nursing executive committees. First, reiterative education. Patients grasp at straws and ignore possible adverse outcomes when they think there is a chance they can be better, have less pain and gain restorative function. Even when risks or percentages are discussed, there is an expectation and entitlement that the patient (and by extension their family) will never be affected by an adverse outcome or complication and will always prevail against the odds. We have a saying in surgery – "the informed consent keeps you out of jail for assault, it doesn't protect you from liability". So, with unexpected events, everyone involved requires high contact and frequent focused education. Waiting for a plaintiff's attorney to regurgitate their 'discovery,' in which every arcane piece of information is presented publicly to impugn a hospital, provider or nurse, (most of which has nothing to do with the case) is a very bad strategy.

A neutral evaluator with access to specialty consultation establishing a pre-dispute quick response 'peer review' would listen to the issues, patient complaints and perspectives, the treating provider's opinions, and then quickly discuss the perceived mistake in a closed session with all affected parties. The treating provider must attend as part of their credentialing requirements. This fosters communication, empathy and understanding.

As a neurosurgeon this was enormously helpful in my surgical practice. No matter how much the clinician attempts to explain issues to patients, there were always unrealistic expectations, particularly with family members. People become quite vindictive when they don't get "the results they paid for." Communication through a neutral third-party stymie's animosity.

Secondly, the evaluation, intervention and remediation must be kept within the medical community. The litigation process is public and acrimonious and there is no presumption of innocence for the healthcare team. A public accusation universally results in simultaneous blame and permanent distrust between all parties. This is not limited to providers and the disaffected patient. Plaintiff lawyers revel in the finger pointing between providers, as they add zeros to their monetary award. Unfortunately, any threat of adverse action causes a profound reflexive defensive position that further alienates providers from their peer support mechanisms. Therefore, coercing a provider under attack to offer an empathetic apology and work through the quality assurance process becomes an insurmountable task.

One pragmatic solution involves separation of the action (problem) from the person (provider) and alleviating the healthcare team from shame while preventing the community from ostracizing the providers. Early ADR intervention concentrates on system mistakes that allowed an error to occur and supports a provider's acknowledgement of errors in judgement, errors of omission or commission, all without devaluing the overall contribution the provider makes to the medical community. Within the confines of the peer review process, providers should receive opportunities to identify mistakes, provide a safe forum to take responsibility and participate in private resolutions. Dragging healthcare providers into the public eye is counterproductive and what the plaintiff's bar and society do not understand is that the internal peer review process and hospital credentialing oversight committees are purposefully draconian. Repeat offenders, in a functioning system, lose their privileges and possibly license long before public censure intervenes.

Lastly, tort education for all parties by the ADR specialist. Litigation pays the lawyers and experts first and the victims get the leftovers. With a 40% contingency fee plus costs of prosecution, including experts charging five to six figures, injured parties receive far less than they believe utilizing the standard court system. Community needs considering safety, an apology, and elimination of financial burden to fix a problem, are never achieved through litigation. The ADR process would reallocate a settlement to the victim and dramatically reduce the "valuation" of those settlements. Although plaintiff attorney's favorite key stroke are the zeros they keep adding onto the claim for damages, the actual court system, awards, judgments and settlements do not respond in kind. So, at the front end, the ADR specialist can educate the patient/potential plaintiff that if they choose an arduous fight, they may receive money for damages, but statistics show that reasonably good plaintiff's lawyers take only 4-6% of the cases brought to them, after obtaining expert reviews. Of that group they process 30-40% by making a claim against the provider or hospital. Factually, survey of why patients sue their providers demonstrate that 37% say they would have been satisfied if they received an honest apology as well as a promise to not allow the mistake to happen again. In addition, 24% of people felt their provider lied or were dishonest in some way. Another 20% sued because they were frustrated that no one would explain what occurred after an adverse outcome and 20% indicated they wanted to prevent a similar issue from affecting someone else. As every insurance carrier will confirm, 33% of people sue their provider because they were instructed to by another party, often a competitor provider group.

Only 25% of plaintiff's surveyed reported their primary motivator was for money. Patients essentially want to know what happened and why, how it will affect their health and how errors can be avoided in the future. Patient also want an apology and not suffer financially because of a provider's error.

Based upon these statistics, an ADR professional should be concentrating on all cases of disgruntled patients and families upset and misinformed that they were victims of medical negligence. Even though 94-96% may never convince a lawyer to take their case, that large number of disaffected people wreak havoc on the valued atmosphere of collaborative healthcare. An effective ADR system within a hospital would encourage investigation of every complaint and issue. This is not just a quick assessment to determine if the hospital or provider has liability exposure. Instead, a root cause analysis of each complaint considering all perspectives will assure attention to a systematic conflict resolution philosophy that institutionally embraces quality improvement, provider satisfaction and optimal patient experience.

The medical ADR specialists assists providers.

Research suggests that after a medical error, patients and family members want to receive a detailed explanation of what happened and why it happened, want to know how the problem will be corrected and future errors prevented, and want to receive an apology. These goals seldom match physician behavior when unexpected clinical outcomes occur. Physicians frequently avoid conversations with the patient and patient's family about what actually occurred and rarely apologize, even empathetically. If our goal is to strengthen the provider-patient relationship, practitioners must cognitively strive to suppress their defensive posture and embrace the collaborative and candid communication exemplified by interest-based mediation. The conversation must extend beyond the exam room and encircle associate care providers, discussing patient safety-oriented issues and encouraging problem solving input. Any adverse outcomes analyzed by root cause discovery, should impact changes in hospital policy or procedure. These modifications should be discussed with patients and families experiencing the inciting event.

Current research demonstrates resistance and limited referral to mediators who use interest-based techniques to resolve medical malpractice lawsuits. The cases that are referred generally occur because of liability exposure, cases considered defensible in court but possibly at risk for a plaintiff verdict, and referrals because plaintiff and defense had significant differing valuation of the case. As litigation shifts toward dispute resolution systems, interest-based mediation presents opportunity to settle cases early in the claim. Judicial settlement conferences usually occur late and on the eve of trial when all parties are angry and polarized. When appropriate, early mediated settlements compensates plaintiffs and avoids costly prolonged discovery as well as the emotional toll on the providers who cannot help but to perseverate on the events causing the claim. Early settlement spares both patients and provider a brutal and emotionally draining process. In addition, system errors that caused or impacted the actual harm are identified and corrected quickly, improving patient safety.

Providers themselves can advocate for early mediation even when a case is defensible, as the framework provides early opportunities to communicate with the patient, now adversary. By utilizing interest-based techniques, research demonstrates that plaintiffs have dismissed or abandon their claims once they receive explanation and an apology. The author experienced this on several occasions as an expert witness in neurosurgery malpractice claims and as a provider ADR expert. Therefore, the author recommends that any provider accused of negligence to aggressively pursue a defense expert witness early in discovery and demand an interest-based mediation once the expert's report supports the care provided. Defense counsel will recommend waiting on these actions but disregard this advice. A proactive provider who communicates with his insurance company and demands these early steps is much better off than following litigation historical procedure. Be cautious in communication with potential experts as any direct communication by phone, email or hard copy is discoverable. Research potential experts with simple inquiry and instruct defense counsel to follow up with direct communication to the potential pool of candidates. These actions dramatically decrease frivolous or weak claims even with adverse care results.

For obscure reasons lawyers, especially on the defense side, are resistant to early interest-based mediation. Per the rules of ethics and American bar association directive in 2006 however, decisions about mediation must be made jointly by lawyers and clients. In reality, most providers merely follow all of their attorney's advice in fear that to disagree, they would be abandon. The provider acquiesces to the lawyers experience to direct the entire process. Although communication, rules of evidence and legal procedure are reserved for the advocate, a provider should not abdicate personal responsibility and divest from the proceedings. Despite the visceral pain from litigation, providers must reframe the experience and strengthen their resolve, actively participating throughout any malpractice claim.

The experienced provider recognizes the benefit to early management using the techniques suggest in this writing. At early mediation, the provider does not have to authorize a demanded financial settlement. In addition, this early neutral evaluation with mediation does not prevent separate judicial mediation later in the case. As Liebman and Hyman confirmed in 2005, lawyers who declined to mediate early did so stating they had not completed adequate discovery. These authors pointed out, these litigators 'may have fallen into the trap of confusing the amount of information required to value a case with the greater amount of information required to prove a case at trial.' Studies of lawyers who were skeptical of early interest-based mediation but participated in the process, demonstrates a very high approval rate and a change to their practices.

Oddly providers resist open communication and often refuse to participate in empathetic conferences with patients and families following adverse events. The same studies demonstrating early interest-based mediation benefitting a defense position, but found that most were performed without provider participation. That extreme position is a mistake. Studies show that defense lawyers who explain away a provider's nonparticipation, run the risk of discounting the value of early mediation and dismiss as insignificant the needs of both plaintiff and provider. As Rowe noted in 2004, providers experience emotional needs after a patient has been harmed by medical care and a provider involved in early interest-based mediation assists them in coping with feelings of guilt or remorse.

Unfortunately, lawyers continue to view mediation through a distributive and evaluative lens, focused on money. Defense counsel fails to understand the second victim syndrome of their distraught provider whose needs might be met by early mediation. Hyman wrote that successful malpractice mediation requires communication with patients and their families following an adverse event or medical error; a full apology when appropriate or an empathetic apology that demonstrates concern for the patient without accepting responsibility if an error did not occur; and if negligence did occur, the commitment to learn from errors and bad outcomes. The provider, not his lawyer must participate and represent themselves with directness, authenticity, and empathy.

Early interests-based mediations provide opportunity for both parties, the defendant provider and the plaintiff patient to be heard and have their concerns and feelings acknowledged. Providers and hospital leaders often fail to appreciate the value of seeking information from patients and families after an error or adverse event, even though this should contribute to improved processes. Levinson demonstrated that effective communication between providers, patients, and family members is the essential element to maintaining identity-based trust and avoiding litigation.

Providers should recall that mediation is confidential and communication in mediation is not discoverable, so a full apology offered in interest-based mediation in front of a plaintiff's lawyer is not discoverable or admissible under rules of evidence if litigation proceeds. In fact, if a plaintiff lawyer asks the provider in subsequent deposition or at trial if he ever apologized for his negligent error (based upon the mediation conversation), defense has immediate grounds to ask for a defense verdict from the judge and then file a grievance against the plaintiff's lawyer with their state bar association. The author witnessed these events and was happy to hear the medical malpractice plaintiff turned her claim against her own unethical lawyer and succeeded with a substantial verdict against him for this behavior.

Recent state laws encourage disclosure of medical errors, although as Shapiro pointed out in 2008, disclosure programs are sporadically implemented and are often resisted by providers, insurers, lawyers, risk managers, and hospital executives. The primary hurdle appears to be the need to coerce providers to improve communication. Surveys demonstrate providers expect to delegate responsibility for communicating with patients to risk managers and hospital lawyers. The same surveys show that non-providers who did not participate in the patient's care lack knowledge and credibility.

One difficulty is that insurance representatives restrict communication between their insured provider and the potential plaintiff early following adverse events. Factually, if providers review their insurance policy, they will likely discover terminology that restricts them from a full apology, lest their insurer reject the claim because the provider breeched the contract. In addition, hospital credentialing may restrict a provider from honest communication following an adverse event. These situations are common, and all providers are encouraged to review these critical practice documents and act to address these issues with companies and hospitals who impose archaic rules proven ineffective at warding off litigation claims. In the end, the providers reputation and ability to practice is at greatest risk, despite obligations to abide by these punitive contracts.

As Liebman and Hyman point out, 'early interest-based mediation offers significant economic and noneconomic benefits to parties to a medical malpractice suit and to society in general.' This author supports their preposition that providers must participate in these processes as key stakeholders would in any mediation.

In addition, medical decision makers, hospital executives, and malpractice insurers must reframe their perception of the tort system enough to view medical mistakes and adverse outcomes as learning opportunities, embracing the concept of early co-mediation using legally trained and medically trained ADR experts, to solve problems, show compassion, and improve care. The era of strictly distributive evaluative mediation fixated only on liability and monetary value or limited to lawyer-to-lawyer negotiations has reached its twilight.

When hospital systems support and embrace the sophisticated professional advocacy of a medically trained ADR expert, the availability and benefits must publicize the values and goals of this endeavor. The ADR must implement programs designed to improve communication, support collegiality, and avoid adverse patient incidents. Safety and quality of healthcare delivery are only part of the ADR mission. Empowering individuals with tools to settle disputes, premeditated sessions with key stakeholders addressing potential conflicts, and a responsive intervention even in minor disputes endears the ADR specialist to the medical staff.

Hospitals and large clinic systems are desperate for an organized high-profile conflict resolution system. Development of these formal process with access available through phone, email, text or anonymously are offered throughout the organization. Repetition is critical and successful dispute resolutions, redacting names and departments to avoid identification, must be shared throughout the clinical environment. Although each participant views their problems as unique and never been tested, that is rarely the case.

Reviewing the facts and process around topics, with strategies and potential solutions, encourages the healthcare worker to address similar situations themselves. The complex integrated system is self-learning and self-improving, quelling turbulence at the lowest possible point of distress.

Healthcare systems are traditionally hierarchical and vertically integrated, where education defines authority, however authority doesn't necessarily recognize responsibility. There are significant opportunities as an ADR healthcare expert to sympathetically disrupt the traditional authoritarian approaches predominant in organized medicine, utilizing communication and negotiation strategies that respect the psychosocial dynamics of integrative and collaborative team work. Importantly, the role of ADR confidant must execute services as a neutral independent that will not report conversations to the hospitals legal department or maintain insider information that administrators could leverage against the doctor or nurse in future negotiations. Providers are often rightfully wary and distrustful of hospital administrations.

ADR healthcare professionals must work to establish trust and confidence even with disruptive or high conflict personalities before a stressful situation arises. Providers must accept the directive and support of the ADR facilitator/mediator/coach first, when not under duress, to improve both consultation, education and functional outcome when a specific conflict arises. The perception that the ADR role as strictly another administrative position controlled by non-providers, with only the hospital's interest at heart, must be dispelled. Anyone assuming an ADR role must work diligently and present their transparent methods of intervention while guarding exclusive conversations as privileged and sacrosanct.

The author constantly discovers that most individuals in the healthcare system lack insight into formal dispute resolution process. Providers can only benefit from skills in strategic negotiation, all facilitated through the ADR office. In the author's role as consultant, a significant amount of time is managing dispositional provider personalities that are claiming and blaming opposing individuals, when these providers are offered the opportunity to parley and benefit from a facilitated or mediated dialogue, they are reticent and embarrassed. The process is so foreign to the traditional discourse paradigms that exist, they fear losing control.

Like most organizations, the hospital environment is functionally dysfunctional and yet, goals are met, and patients are cared for, even when emotions run high with anger and resentment, rumbling precariously just below the surface for many providers. Healthcare practitioners resist opportunities to work through their stressful and adverse experiences and fear exploring mutual interests with their adversaries. Providers have yet to appreciate the availability and benefits an ADR medical professional can provide to their practice.

Negotiations, mediations and facilitations are tough work. As a third-party intermediary, mounting frustration can affect identification of adequate, if not optimal solutions. When reticent and unwilling parties appear to waste time and dismiss the mediator's efforts, the third-party negotiator might fall prey to the negotiators dilemma (Lax 1992), unwilling to yield to an acceptable outcome. Not uncommon, type-A personality providers default to hard positional stances once circular arguments disrupt negotiation. Opponents demonstrate unwillingness to respect each other's contributions during conversation. Quickly parties are guilty of competitive demands and polarize away from any collaborative agreement.

This shift toward a competitive style exposes traditional provider bias that discounts the opponent's interests, encouraging escalating conflict and disregards their opponents status and needs. Providers are enraged when their adversary dismisses the time value and significance of the negotiations themselves or is uninterested and ill prepared for the negotiation. In these instances, the ADR witnesses one party rush to conclude (and win) the negotiation, pressing a victory blitzkrieg assault that eventually concentrates on subjugation and dismissal of the opponents interests. These emotionally driven behaviors should be expected, and the ADR must be prepared to intercede before the exchange becomes toxic.

A Case of maturing ADR influence.

An example of a maturing and effective dispute management system is studies at the Kaiser Permanente Healthcare Maintenance Organization. The organization employs ombudsman in the HCOM (healthcare ombudsman) position in a parallel pathway to risk management. The position is independently administered, and all conversations and disclosures are confidential, protected from litigation discovery. Their respected and published medical ADR persona, HCOM Tarrant, paraphrases her role as a healthcare ADR professional, 'I assist patients and providers by helping them to work together to address their needs and interests. This includes acting to fairly resolve healthcare issues, disputes and conflicts by acting as a neutral, independent and confidential resource for patients, families and providers. It is the job of the HCOM to understand the dynamics of patient-provider communication and the relational aspects of dispute resolution.' The intervention facilitates doctor-patient relationships through communication management particularly when adverse outcomes leave families distressed and vulnerable.

The HCOM is recognized and easily accessible by any provider in the Kaiser system and responds quickly to concerns confidentially disclosed by any medical team member. Annually, HCOM training

177

includes seminars from Professor Gerald Monk of San Diego State University whose concentrated review instructs the new HCOM to 'breathe ... and remember that even though you can't control the outcome, everything you do can help move the people and the situation toward healing.' The HCOM training targets employees with very little medical education.

The new HCOM, like every ADR professional starting their career, is reminded that as the third-party observer to conflicts, emotions expressed toward them are often displaced aggression between parties in conflict. This is ubiquitous across the coaching, facilitator and mediator experience for healthcare ADR specialists. The person emotionally venting on a third-party sees the mediator as a safe target and often transfers the frustration of the dispute with unbridled intensity. Often the empathetic third-party is a calming influence, actively listening and slowly re-framing the perspective, providing insight when available.

The HCOM is coached to stay curious, take time for themselves, to regroup their thoughts, stay centered, and not succumb to personal outbursts. Inexperience is not ignorance and 'amid turbulent emotions and adversarial encounters, stay grounded in the knowledge that your calming presence with, as much as your words, have the power to heal and transform this encounter.' In addition, sage word of advice remind ever conflict manager to hear everyone's experience before assuming what actually caused the conflict. Head the words of wisdom: 'Promise little. Deliver Much., but don't own the outcome.'

Tasks for the ADR Healthcare specialist

1. Develop skill sets in narrative communication as preventive maintenance for professional relationships. Identify the common scenario of misconception, miscommunication, and dispositional claims between healthcare providers in the hierarchical system that create the conflicts and expose the flaws and potential solutions of these adversarial positions.

2. Introduce and encourage professional collegiality training. Establish a role modeling benchmark to emulate, rewarding professionalism for the healthcare provider. Utilize coaching programs to emphasize skills in congeniality and reinforcing safety behavior while trying to influence a cultural shift away from totalitarian hierarchical behavior and toward a team's first approach. The goal is to eliminate the toxic work place perception that occurs when individuals are belittled and chastised. Respectful discourse can be taught.

3. Establish an efficient communication platform between providers to convey critical information to avoid mistakes. A common successful methodology is the "S bar" program, adopted by hospital systems throughout the world. S-Bar stands for: 'Situation, Background, Assessment, Recommendation'; a technique to facilitate prompt and appropriate communication. Do not assume any system is being effectively administered. Take the responsibility to test the system for flaws, errors or inefficient use. Encourage systematic repetition by mock practice scenarios that everyone in the healthcare system must complete. No exceptions.

4. The organization concentrates on measurable metrics related to identification of concern that is reproducible, such as the emergent STOP program when a team member suspects an error or adverse event is underway. 'Stop the Line' is a VA-wide initiative that empowers VHA employees to speak up immediately if they see a risk to patient safety. The model encourages employees to report behaviors, action, or inaction that might result in errors or patient harm. Confirm an accurate incident report details the issue, what actions influenced the error, and perform a root cause analysis of significant events. Include multiple parties such as the chief medical officer, chief nursing officer, floor and

department managers, risk management, the parties in conflict, human resources with their advocate, and department chairs as needed.

5. An establish chain of command that weighs the incidents impact on individuals, the institution and ultimately patient safety. These fourth-party system stakeholders are tasked to recognize and discuss corrective actions to be adopted by the system.

    a. Parties are defined: first and second party are the conflict principals; third-party is the active dispute manager; fourth party are the stakeholders responsible for systems design; Fifth party is the unaffiliated general population.

6. Utilize continuing education to expand both your ADR training while identifying pathways and programs that prove useful resources to the institution. The Healthcare Professional Institute and their "Safety first class" is an example. As a consultant, the author often recommends training modules for all healthcare providers, mandatory for employees and required to maintain provider credentialing.

7. The ADR should encourage, monitor and participate in every program designed to improve patient care communication and address care delivery difficulties. These are often programmed as daily patient huddles, weekly team building bedside rounds, and monthly administrative opportunities where staff members use negotiation skills to defuse mock conflicts. Programs that maintain dispute identification and management techniques should be developed and steadily rolled out without interfering with providers busy clinical schedule.

8. Develop a mass communication system at the organizational level, updating staff on events and dispelling rumors and hearsay when critical issues arise. Keep vested parties informed. Error recognition, conflict and recovery with resolution, are shared with staff and vital for emotional health.

9. Following a sentinel events (severe patient injury or death), the ADR professional must participate in the sophisticated analysis working closely with the risk management department. After the root cause analysis, the ADR specialist can be an excellent buffer during difficult system adjustments dictated to the medical staff. The ADR must learn to deliver results framed as opportunities where

medical and nursing providers identify and develop consensus agreement on how to modify care pathways to prevent future similar events. Individuals involved must be included in a non-blaming method of incident management and improvement.

10. The ADR skill set does not stop at the emergency room door. Individual practices require outpatient support. ADR personnel must be available to the providers to remain consistent with their approach to communication and safety in the healthcare settings. The critical extension is ignored in most institutions. If practices are not consistent in both outpatient and inpatient behavior, the systems will falter and fail.

11. Focus on healthcare provider wellness and professional support during adverse events. Providers are pillorized and expected to remain stoic when under stress and attack. Issues such as peer reviews, medical board inquiry and especially litigations are so distracting that statistics show the providers will make additional mistakes during those times. Preoccupation with medical malpractice disputes causes additional errors and higher subsequent claim statistics. This should not happen. We can avoid this safety issue and help heal the emotional and psychological torment of our

most valuable assets – the healthcare provider. Be sure there are confidential opportunities for the providers to vent, share their fears and maintain that rapport well after an event has concluded. Self-improvement psychological counseling are stigmatized by providers, so the ADR healthcare trained professional serves as an excellent resource for distressed practitioners.

12. Convince the organization that medically trained ADR services are critical to strategic operations. Gaining traction in any organization or applying for the position of ADR specialist in an uneducated medical practice can be difficult. The author suggests utilizing those negotiating skills to pitch the position in a frame that demonstrates ADR as a value-added service to the organization. Train first, then offer the spectrum of mediation services for disputes your organization finds challenging to its operational success. Point out that conflicting parties consume valuable resources and detract from the hospital's core mission and commerce. Illustrate the value offered by a healthcare trained provider with expertise in the field of ADR.

As the text demonstrates, there is a spectrum of conflict management interventional approaches. In the field of mediation, the professional consultant will often default to a style they find applicable to the engagement, based upon the disputing party's relationships and goals. A new ADR will hone their skills by researching and resolving the immediate disputes plaguing the system, offering congenial and professional future relationships between staff, patients and administration. The ADR remains focused on deliverable services representing the fundamental role of facilitation and mediation, as an expert managing communication, and develops unique exchange channels between opponents. An ADR should be present to manage the group dynamics of people in conflict. Conflict manager maintains a lean forward agenda to discover the foundations of the dispute, exploring interests, needs and objectives for all parties embroiled in any given argument.

The ADR must process information with critical reframing of positional declarations to alter the effective narrative voice. The ADR's greatest contribution to the systems dispute management will be to neutralize the emotional and recalcitrant extremes by facilitating understanding and empathy between adversaries. A healthcare trained ADR professional's breath of knowledge enables the frequent and necessary shift in approach and orientation to a dispute, from evaluative to facilitative interest-based counselor, discovering opportunities to micromanage long-term relationships using a transformative storyline, demonstrating to the parties a vision of valuable future collaborative.

Since most administrators, staff and providers see conflict as a pain point and desire immediate, even sub optimal resolution, the ADR utilizes the conflict as an educational opportunity, applying appreciative inquiry to generalize the reasons behind the conflict. Through educational efforts in the organization, the ADR assists in a broad and introspective understanding of causation behind each conflict and establishes a process toward resolution, developing a blueprint for successful management of similar future disputes.

The ADR must always remind superiors and parties that not every conflict will be resolved and although the ADR remains dedicated to that goal, at the very least a mediation produces a rich understanding and communication of the issues between adverse parties. The ADR role remains committed to assist the parties while acting neutral as an administrative facilitator. The ADR must continually establish boundaries that rejects any coercion or heavy-handed influence to favor one 'side.' The ADR often strives to balance the power differential between individuals, particularly when education separates roles in the healthcare hierarchy. An imperative in any dispute management system is institutional confirmation that parties in conflict, who have less power than the organization, will not face sanction, fear retribution, or retaliation for voicing their opinions, desires and interests. The ADR specialist has an ethical obligation to ratify this commitment from senior staff and administrators.

In summary, the medically trained ADR specialist can broker business disputes, address staff interpersonal conflicts, deal with high conflict persons in power positions, assume an Ombudsman role that develops and participates in disclosures of adverse events, work with risk management developing and implementing system wide dispute resolution education and co-mediate with a legal counterpart, elective and court ordered prelitigation tort actions.

Chapter Eight

Established models as guidelines for conflict management systems

There are several Models referenced here for the reader to explore. These are each variations on the same ADR theme. These models assist the new ADR professional, utilizing an established model as a direction to gain institutional support. The appendix references these models for expanded study. Systems include the *Rush Model*, in which two attorneys provide mediation services during disputes; the *Veterans Administration (VA) model*, advocating for full and immediate disclosure after an event. In the VA approach, following rapid internal evaluation, the ombudsman, risk management and a VA legal representative attempt to negotiate fair compensation and ensures corrective action if mistakes were made by the medical personnel; The *University of Michigan model* quickly evaluates and fairly compensate unreasonable medical care causing injury, but importantly demands an objective evaluation and a strong defense for frivolous claims; the *Pew model* and *Internal neutral mediator model* both support a robust ADR specialist approach to patient – provider conflict through objective assessment, needs evaluation, education and empathetic apology (apology without admitting liability or error) for claims without medical negligence. There are ADR solutions in place to quickly close a claim when errors of omission or commission did occur resulting in medicine below the standards of care. A professional assuming the helm of a conflict engagement system might choose to expand on these models, focusing on patient-provider interactions, system education for the entire medical complex, and then open to the dynamic interchange within every organization which constantly experiences friction and inefficiency because of unresolved conflict.

Another option, the *consensus model* is defined by the participants finding unity in solutions even if they do not unanimously agree with every facet of the opinion or plan. Consensus is intended to consider diverse perspectives, validating the efforts and worth of each participant's point of view. The model requires each participant assume ultimate responsibility for the overall agreed opinion of the collective. In addition, the participant must not acquiesce to proposals they consider significantly faulty and must block proposals they strongly disagree with. Often agreements are elusive and reticent positioning by key persons rejecting a consensus opinion is frustrating for the ADR, as these individuals may not offer constructive suggestions as viable alternatives. Ghais writes on extreme facilitation, or facilitation in extremely challenging conditions, providing practical and strategic suggestions for the ADR determined to ensure an effective managed resolution to conflicts with these types of stakeholders. The skills recommended are assessment, convening, contracting, and process design. These progressive stages are: assessment allowing the facilitator to immediately understand the groups goals, cultures and objectives; the convening step determines who are the authorities who have a vested interest in the process, so the ADR can bring them to the table; the contracting phase requires the facilitator to outline the informal and formal agreement and work effort required to accomplish the tasks at hand; and the process design phase, which is critical to the facilitators successful management of the engagement, providing a flexible procedural mechanism and paradigm for the group to define, stay on task, and finally accomplish its strategic goals.

Carlson writes about key components for improving group's effectiveness through consensus building, including determining a clear and shared vision between group members; generating a supportive culture that suspends judgment and allows free flow of targeted ideas; rewards participants who consistently contribute to the objective analysis and problem solving steps required for consensus opinion identification; open and detailed information sharing, including feedback about performance; training and consultation to secure a shared power participation; supportive technology, material resources and a comfortable adequate physical environment to stimulate the exchange. One conflict management model, the *complex theory modeling and collaborative design*, mimics sophisticated system software design that requires logic inferences based upon optimal outcomes, defined by established positions. The group interaction specifically demands a collaborative information gathering environment to consider learning as a social process, incorporating 'multiple distinguishable phases that constitute a cycle of personal and social knowledge-building.' The theory, advocated by Gerry Stahl, allows us to replace the computer modeling interface with the facilitator role. The process suggests that the group will effectively manage increasingly complex questions during negotiations as their interaction secures a sophisticated understanding of each other's needs and interests.

This model is similar to the *social learning model* if discourse and communication is 'relatively free of hidden agendas, power struggles and un-discussed prejudices.' As a null hypothesis for logic testing, one assumes that negotiation from positional perspectives will not result in a consensus opinion and there will be no new knowledge gained causing negotiations to fail. Logic theory states that failure will occur only when one or more parties demand a set of circumstances that their opponents consider extreme, rejecting a compromise solution that should yield mutual gain. To avoid the null outcome, this model requires the facilitator to create an exchange network that ensures effective communication, demonstrating social interaction skills such as turn-taking, repair of misunderstandings, rhetorical persuasion, and interactive arguing between negotiating parties. The knowledge based integrative design calls for consideration of positional sides but facilitates comparison viewpoints, 'in which one can view and contrast alternative perspectives and adopt or adapt ideas from other people's perspectives.' The comparison evaluations aggregates ideas from distributive opposite demands and provides the structure to contrast the merits and contentions of each opinion in a discussion forum.

Critical to consensus building, subsequent buy-in and adaptation of solutions throughout the system requires learning from the dynamic interactive communication interchange, stimulating people to consider and respond to alternative proposals. Key stakeholders around a negotiating table will reveal over-lapping positional interests, discuss concessions and ultimately build consensus. According to Bryson, this model encourages 'discourse to introduce competing organizations (or individuals) to merge into a new entity (relationship) to handle problems through their shared authority and capabilities.' Critical to the outcome are coordinated initiatives and shared power, designed to pool resources and skills to address specific needs.

Bryson further discusses the optimal environment for a facilitator to encourage a successful negotiation. He reminds the third-party coordinator that stakeholders will be influenced by hidden agendas or stressors and that collaborators are subject to both 'competitive and institutional pressures that significantly affect ...their long-term sustainability.' The aggregate of individuals within a medical system function as a social collective with normative behavior, legal, and regulatory elements dictating how the organization thinks and performs. These rules bind viewpoints and stymie potential new perspectives, dictating behavior and influencing negotiations disproportionally with positional demands. Often a distributive requirement by one side escapes understanding by the opposition party. In addition, past or collateral relationships impact the network effect influencing the current negotiation. In other words, for one party to accept a new facilitated relationship, a stakeholder must overcome their reticence as the new collaboration will have access and a subsequent ripple effect across past relationships for each party. Thus, the stakeholder reaching an agreed compromised solution becomes the interloper or ambassador that introduces the new member to established networks. Therefore, the risks are high for each party, protecting their social and professional connections exposed at the bargaining conference.

The facilitator must consider several critical steps required to orchestrate a successful negotiation paradigm for this group. The process requires achieving benchmarks before moving forward. The pivot points include forging initial agreements (both informal and formal), building leadership amongst group members, building legitimacy for the outcome of the collaborative exercise, building trust between positional future partners in the venture, managing conflict by anticipating current and future hurdles while negotiating immediate and potential solutions. The goals for facilitative intervention include: formal agreements that consider overall purpose, commitment, dedicated resources, establishing recognized and dependable leadership, a reproducible decision-making structure, and flexibility for the decision makers to adapt to changing conditions which call for quick decisions and not prolonged bureaucratic delays. Key stakeholders must collaborate with those implementing the solutions to assure commitment to negotiated solutions.

These consensus collaborations are more likely to succeed when they have steadfast sponsors and effective champions that provide leadership during negotiations and act as resources once agreements are reached. Between the two sides of dispositional negotiators, the facilitator must investigate opportunities for trust building. Trusting relationships are often depicted as the essence of collaboration. These relationships facilitate the work of collaboration and bind the design together. Distrust compromises interpersonal behavior, confidence in organizational competence and performance, and threatens the common bond and perception of goodwill that group consensus represents. As Bryson points out, trusting relationships are: 'Paradoxically, they are both the lubricant and the glue' that creates alliances.

The facilitative ADR professional assumes the advocate responsibility as conflict manager and therefore the interloper between opponents. The ADR prioritizes agenda items and expectations that parties bring to a negotiation, from perspectives on strategies and tactics to control over the collaboration's work product. The facilitator understands that less powerful partners often require assurance that their interests are being considered. An ADR expert who can neutralize the power differentials will manage conflict effectively and provide long term structure to the group, assisting future conflict management.

The collaborative consensus design integrates elements of cooperative efforts with the *computer logic model* proposed by Da Yang. Here, a facilitator's goals and interests are foundational and enacted as a step wise functional structure, designed to illicit key stake holder participation and dedication. The facilitator follows a sequence of steps and instructions to guide the parties working out mutually satisfactory requirements to meet their goals. During each step, the facilitator offers a variety of project tools designed to generate, organize, and evaluate concepts and new information. This model is an excellent outline for a new medical ADR attempting mediation efforts. Specifically, Da Yang describes the process as:

1. Identify and engage all stakeholders and hold pre-meeting caucus with each client to completely understand their operational significance to the negotiation and outcome control of the negotiations. Each important stakeholder becomes a 'Shaper and Personal Knowledge Contributor (PKC).'

2. The project continues with the stakeholder's initial meeting which functions as the first collaborative learning process as the facilitator executes specific practices.
   a. The facilitator introduces their role as the learning coordinator.
   b. The meetings begin by defining learning objectives developed by consensus.
   c. Stakeholders utilize appreciative inquiry discovering past successes of collaborative partnerships and focus on the methodologies for successful conditions (win conditions, issues, options, and agreements).

3. Assessment, goal review and progress report with accountability objectives are defined, summarizing each successful learning objective and identifying future needs.

4. Review and expand negotiation topics which are organized according to consensus priority to guide and focus the stakeholder negotiation. This maintains organized information flow between opponents and minimizes tangential conversations that subvert attention from critical topics and goals.

5. The process of brainstorming ideas and initiatives all converge on win-win conditions for both parties, keeping in mind the ultimate objective. In healthcare, core needs permeate all negotiations and stakeholders are often reminded their work is framed by delivery of expert and efficient healthcare.

6. Perform a review of consensus contracts and conditions using a multi-criteria evaluation to rate each 'win' condition along two measures: business importance and ease of realization. This step provides opportunity to challenge or potentially to block an initiative and this encourages non-threatening open debate as to the merits of specific positions and their impact on the global negotiations.

7. Through discourse, resolve differences. Conflicts arise, followed by solutions that benchmark and create the structure for a working design used in subsequent negotiations. Achieving early consensus on minimally debated issues demonstrates the potential of collaboration. Harder issues to agree upon are passed into the 'funnel theory of discourse.' The remaining conditional agreements or outright rejections are then negotiated, and positional compromise is far easier to accomplish as opponents recognize their counter's needs and offer good faith considerations when there is productive exchange.

8. The facilitator ensures the solutions are disseminated throughout the hospital system utilizing multiple channels of asynchronous communication (a single email or newsletter post is not adequate to ensure solutions are adopted by the system). What follows is a continuous refinement stage adapting to the evolving nature of requirements for implementation. The facilitator is responsible for systems learning and the stakeholders continue to ensure the system accepts and acts upon the negotiated solutions.

9. Finally, the interest-based mediator style favors an integrative mutually beneficial solution-oriented approach.

The *computational logic theory* mirrors the collapsed design of the Tuckman and Dimock *group dynamic models* which provide the medical ADR with a framework to ensure effective contract negotiations. Here the facilitator defines the parameters to inspire the vision statement or the 'motivating task' that assumes a null hypothesis: 'task A cannot be accomplished.' Logic and game theory disproves the hypothesis utilizing appreciative design which supports algorithms that generate functional data solutions tied to specific tasks. In our healthcare facilitators case, the efforts is focused on a specific contracting negotiation and agreement. This model requires that fundamental interactions use predictability measures if the group acts rationally. It assumes that basic human requirements of inclusion, control and relationships are met during stakeholder pathway mental mapping.

The psychometric adaption proposed by Tuckman envisions stepwise progression through functional group interaction where stages of progressive maturation ensure negotiation success. This sociologic model anticipates behavioral human interaction for the "forming, storming, norming and performing stages of group dynamics" and will predict aberrant individual interactions which could potentially block consensus opinion ratification. The facilitator must be responsive and adaptable by establishing a practice pattern which addresses the conflict pressure points. The ADR professional relies upon group discussion between those in consensus and the opposing dissenting voices during every negotiation.

The model requires progressive compromise between agents followed by formalized agreements when they occur and recommends delayed negotiation for topics in contention. Following this paradigm, the *corollary logic pareto agreement model* predicts a high percentage of negotiated agreements, contract consensus and only a small pool of holdout topics or issues. The group would define issues to be 'carved out' and discussed at subsequent meetings.

Tuckman's detailed 'Forming, Storming, Norming, and Performing' model and are effective to build consensus amongst a like-minded group whose goals, values and agreed upon mission objectives are well articulated in the forming or assessment stages of group collaboration. The ADR anticipates that individuals who are interacting from a cautious and reticent position when sharing their ideas requires a safe, interactive and nonjudgmental environment. The facilitator actively listens and dynamically reframes during group communication, supporting individual perspectives and encouraging brainstorming discourse. Once established, objectives and mission statements motivate key players into the convening and storming phase of open dissection and discussion of positions in order to arrive at the norming phase.

As Gais points out, an effective norming and performing stage must have the structure of detailed contracting to highlight benchmark objectives and ensure the group stays on task, concentrating on the agreed goal statements generated from the early convening stages. The effective group continues to modify and embrace efficiencies in the process design phase that allows maximal performance and successful administration of the group's objectives. Dimock's theory closely correlates with essential group acceptance. Passage through Tuckman's storming stage, arriving at the norming or consensus building stage, supports individual 'inclusion, control and connection.' As Dimock illustrates, a group will be stuck in the storming phase and prevent the facilitation of effective contracting and structure building if '...a group that has not resolved inclusion and control issues is unlikely to develop much in the area of connection.' These models all assume that a successful process occurs only as the group effectively matures through each sequential stage without residual conflict or unresolved contention.

These various integrated models mirror software networking mind map solutions to problem solving. They all identify key stakeholders and use the facilitator to create an organized opportunity to stimulate conversation and identify the essential nature of important issues to collaborate under a common vision. This action creates a new knowledge metric that defines future integrative solutions to this groups disputes and contractual challenges.

Distilling these various themes creates a template for the healthcare ADR expert. Begin with pre-meeting caucus followed by position statement and discussion. Move forward with investigating areas of common need and solutions through focused target subgroups and general meeting of principals. The most productive discussions and opportunities for solutions begin with appreciative inquiry. Solidify early solutions, documenting the progress and filter out the polarizing topics, saving those discussions for subsequent consideration. The facilitator's role in system design, conversation, discourse management, and solution ratification, creates a functional new knowledge set that each party will be compelled, through commitment and participation, to ratify.

These models conclude by affirming that stakeholders return to their respective departments and emphasize that the expanded groups and organizations, whose members were the key stakeholders, adopt the resolutions from negotiation and not renege on ratified agreements. These models foundationally follow interest-based mediation dictum and document these methods as successful guidelines for dispute resolution.

The *logic-based model* for the facilitator to reference will maximize areas of consensus between parties, imposing appreciative design theory of dynamic collaborative group behavior, to arrive at a successful negotiation between disparate party positions. According to Ragone, "it is possible to have many issues negotiated among many parties" however there will likely be hidden agendas because of "the interplay among shifting coalitions: parties can join and act against other parties involved." The facilitator will present bargaining as either a cooperative or non-cooperative game. Theoretically, representatives of each negotiating group are individually rational and unlikely to accept a deal which involves a loss, i.e., a disadvantageous deal. Practically however, the self-interested agents negotiate over a set of resources to obtain an optimal allocation of these resources while maximizing the concessions from their counterpart group.

As a facilitator, our approach uses logic-based negotiation strategies to discover and delineate the space of possible deals or potential agreements; determine the set of rules and methodology this group will utilize through-out negotiations (the negotiation protocol), and supervise negotiation strategy each agent adopts, within the set of rules specified in the negotiation protocol. The logic theory of maximal gain simultaneously achieved for optimal negotiation results dictates that when several items are being negotiated simultaneously, an integrative conclusion allows each issue to assume a different utility or importance score. As collaborative agents we then can define a new reality in the relationship where cooperation providing "more for one party" does not necessarily result in their opponent receiving "less".

There are critical ground rules for the facilitator using a logic-based system, to communicate openly and honestly with all stakeholder participants. Only then can the facilitator, based upon logic driven conclusions, define the optimum solutions from each party. At this point, we as facilitators in consensus discussion with all stakeholders, will outline proposed agreements mutually beneficial for both parties. These agreements maximize both social welfare and individual organizational interests discovered as stakeholder requirements utilizing consensus opinion modeling for an integrative contract solution.

Perhaps the greatest challenge for the medical ADR will be shifting roles and responsibilities in the clinical setting. As the ADR redefines their skills brought to the table during conflict discourse, the ADR toolbox will for some time be foreign and awkward. Frankly, it will always be easier to listen to a clinical story, develop a differential diagnosis and recommend a host of laboratory studies, than it will be to apply psycho-social and communication tactics to define a problem and consider options for cure. For most providers, the clinical experience is no longer an academic exercise but a daily reality. When we choose to reframe our focus and contribution as an ADR professional, as a third-party role facilitator, mediator or coach, we request our peers provide some latitude as we develop these skills. This is quite different than the harsh reality of clinical practice so critical of perceived errors in patient management. The learning will be exponential and progressive as conflict is pervasive, if not insidious.

The author recommends taking solace in the gestalt view and simple fact, that the resultant outcome of dispute resolution is dependent on the parties and not the ADR and when disputants fail to resolve their differences, this does not equate to an incompetent third-party neutral.

Chapter Nine

The Authors Journey from
Healthcare to ADR specialist

As a clinician for 30 years, my professional experience focused on managing the physician-patient relationship. On one hand, I am a scientist and apply all the technical knowledge about disease management, while in the other, a compassionate salesman, convincing often frightened and wary patients and families to trust my skilled hands. Surgery requires informed consent after just a few meetings in the foreign surrounds of the clinic or hospital, while patients ignore or at least suppress their own fears and trepidations natural to these conversations. My skills in negotiation really come from pediatric neurosurgery (as a necessity, not on purpose), for if there is ever a time when conversations require delicate conflict management skills, it is with parents of sick children. Responding appropriately to the quick defensive anger and hostility when the clinical course is not perfect, or even when the diagnosis is poor and the family projects their fury and disbelief onto the healthcare providers, as if we caused the disease. All of these cases require a calm understanding of predictable situational extremes, navigating emotional and visceral hind brain irrational demands, attempting to restore calm and balance.

As a neurosurgeon, I have experienced every type of conflict, disclosure and the process of administrative and tort litigation. The system is so broken, beyond what we fathom. Strained communication between provider and patient is a small portion of the dilemma. The healthcare provider's gauntlet includes painful administrative inquiry and oppression endured from the myriad of regulatory agencies, peers, competitors, foes and law firms. Accusations and attribution errors constantly put providers on their highest guard. I doubt many of us are dispassionate, but the high walls constructed to protect and preserve our emotional sanity suppress expressions of compassion and empathy shielded just to ensure we survive the turmoil of professional clinical practice.

Having practiced ADR skills while a physician, I do have my bias, if not prejudice on effective mediation techniques. There are no absolutes or strict adherence to one theory or method of conflict engagement. A competent and studied ADR professional utilizes a multi-modality approach when dealing with situations and personalities. In fact, regardless of which style a practitioner adopts, each method should be tactically and strategically deployed under the auspices of a capable conflict management practice. Constants in the practice are reflective insight, active listening, and creative engagement, ensuring that the disputants receive the superior services of a facilitator, mediator or arbitrator with depth and breadth of skills to remain flexible and adaptive. When the medical practitioner changes the hat from clinician to ADR practitioner, they must provide elements of transformative, facilitative, and narrative mediation techniques even when the concentration of efforts and desire of litigators calls for evaluative methodology.

As a medical subject matter healthcare expert, litigated disputes requesting my consultation requires direct contact and conversation with paid expert witnesses. These 'hired guns' will either challenge or support the previous medical care provided to a plaintiff. Many experts use propaganda techniques and claim their opinion as authoritative and immutable. Cases hinge on the 'expert' testimony paid for by the plaintiff or defense, where concepts of standards of care, critical to allegations of negligence are often nebulous. Sifting through the bravado, anticipating positional demands, and interpreting the facts and medical records are all required of an effective neutral ADR tort claims co-mediator and co-arbitrator. We wear both medical and legal hats when participating in these disputes.

The authors own technique utilizes an interest-based evaluative design and directive mediation model as a co-mediator and co-arbitrator during litigated healthcare disputes. The effective utilization of evaluative techniques complements any provider's experience and skill set in healthcare delivery. Providers are mentally wired to process information using a scientific and didactic approach. As a consultant and subject matter expert, despite a conflict specialist's fervent desire to explore the psycho-social issues that create conflict, the ADR specialist must address and manage the evaluative aspect that parties request when involved in late phase mediation. Should more negligence disputes request early mediation, styles will shift toward interest-based approaches that minimize evaluative input. Most parties want advice and resolution if they agree to private dispute mediation. Successful mediation must respect the goals of the clients which create the ethical mandate when contracting to provide ADR services.

Currently, emphasis on mediation evaluative approach focuses on a mutually acceptable settlement of the dispute. The mediator investigates the substance of the dispute, medical facts supporting the positions, attempts to de-escalate the conflict through advisory consultation and then determines if consensus on settlement is possible. Injecting interest based themes takes time and effort, often overcoming resistance from lawyers representing parties. That said, structured group discussion prior to demands of monetary settlement during mediation, provides the ADR a perfect opportunity for patient/plaintiff discussion with providers, meeting the goals discussed throughout this text. The ultimate settlement discussions are often simpler as both sides acknowledge the impact of the adverse outcome, humanize their adversary and are empathetic to the impact of the results and conflict on each other's lives. The medical ADR must separate the clinical role and prejudice from the ADR mandate. The ADR is a nonclinical individual assisting parties understanding of all medically related issues and negotiating toward dispute resolution. The medical ADR must supplant one's clinical orientation with an intermediary's impartiality, advocating for a fair and considerate settlement.

The author engages constantly in reflective practice as an ADR medical expert while balancing evaluative and narrative mediation skills. The author receives requests for assistance from all types of providers and their insurance companies seeking to ensure they have a competent and neutral subject matter expert at early and court ordered mediations. As arbitration clauses are enacted, the author is honored to serve the role of subject matter expert on arbitration panels. While participating in the closed-door caucuses, the author recognizes overzealous plaintiffs, enthusiastic and committed to their attribution errors and positional demands. Despite unfavorable statistics, plaintiffs are universally convinced they will prevail with a favorable verdict from litigation. In addition, the provider is usually over enthusiastic about their sound defense. Also, the author's expertise is requested by lawyers, hospitals and courts to provide the same balanced perspective to these processes, independent of the legal bantering seen between lawyer -mediators without deep healthcare knowledge. In practice, the author always reiterates the position requires impartiality, reminding the medical personnel that a perceived error, if compellingly argued by plaintiff's experts, will convince a jury that the plaintiff was negligently treated and injured.

The author spends a considerable amount of time facilitating for providers involved with administrative investigations from medical boards and medical staff committees which prejudices against the provider with harsh critical analysis of medical errors through the peer review process. The author is witness to the impact of inadequate regulations and the damage resultant from systematic mediocre care, however providers are assumed guilty by colleagues and administrative bodies once accused and the provider, despite what their lawyer may tell them, has the burden of proof to successfully argue their care was appropriate.

With the maturation of the information age, patients are savvy consumers before and after treatment. Aggressively challenging suboptimal or poor outcomes is easy with the glut of tort litigation counsel available, even when standard of medical care are met. Disgruntled patients file claims, complain to medical boards, and with the prolonged process of litigation, become entrenched playing the victim's role with dispositional and distributive demands. The patients assume the victim narrative and talk freely to the press, while the provider is cautioned by lawyers and their insurance company to remain silent. Attempting to avert a providers descension into this abyss, the ADR role calls for evaluative input. The author routinely discusses the case (redacting identities), with experts in the field of medicine, factoring in the plaintiff's co-morbid medical issues and examining the details of medical care provided. As such, as a co-mediator, this provider-ADR professional offers perspective on the likelihood of a strong plaintiff or defense argument after personally interviewing each expert witness. In the third-party position, the mediator will, during caucus communication, assess if the plaintiff, as a patient, understood the risks and expectations of the care received as well as ferret out the motivations behind filing a medical malpractice case.

As an ADR specialist, the author is afforded the third person neutral view of an argument as well as the fourth person system or organizations view of the dispute. When studying dysfunctional provider-patient communication, it becomes apparent that tension is a byproduct of a medical macro-climate which breeds anxiety and fear into the providers entrusted with the emergencies of physical and psychological disease directing patients to our door. The author agrees with Chen's assertion that establishing a relationship through integrative design minimizes the chance that adverse outcomes will result in complaints or litigation. ' Not surprisingly, those patients with the strongest relationships to specific primary care physicians ...or have a longstanding relationship with a doctor...have a doctor who knows him or her as a human being.' These relationships diminish claims and misunderstandings and allow the provider relaxed creativity while approaching medical treatment. When that relationship is continually threatened by outside influences that punish the provider, the result is a wary, dispassionate, unsympathetic technician.

Should it ever become necessary to discuss a potential error or complication with treatments, these issues are received as a betrayal of limited trust. The provider should expect anger and retribution by patients and families. This is human nature. Over the years, my intimate interviews with healthcare providers leads me to the simple conclusion that providers are in constant fear for their own professional health and security. Providers feels they are under constant threat and attack. They have limited trust toward their colleagues, administration and patients. Although we desire Maslow's self-actualization in our professions, conflict inevitably prevents us from rising above the quagmire. Encumbered with a constantly reactive and defensive mental state eliminates personal and professional growth and satisfaction. From my own journey, the author considers the role of a sophisticated conflict manager embedded into healthcare systems as a critical need and resource for providers to access, resolving dilemmas and supporting practitioners' desires through collaborative institutional conflict systems design.

As a start, the medical ombudsman provides a pathway for ADR skill adaptation with a recognized job description. These opportunities are available in organizations such as universities, the military medical complex and large HMOs. As the text points out, the ombudsman initial and primary function as previously discussed by Houk and Amerson, is managing empathetic apologies in the healthcare setting. The ombudsman quickly functions as the coordinator between the clinical key stakeholders and identifies the clinical 'Captain of the ship', as well as stakeholder family members, while managing difficult conversations related to adverse events and medical errors. The ADR professional ensures that the provider continues to discuss with the family all information they need to understand and hopefully gain closure following an unanticipated bad outcome. The message must be clear and the ADR professional bridges the provider-patient relationship through advocacy for both parties, maintaining trust and compassion and mitigating against adversarial positioning. This requires constant conversations lead by the conflict manager.

The ADR specialist is always present and provides the clinician with guidelines to improve discourse with a distraught family. As a younger neurosurgeon, I assumed this responsibility in my own practice and never received counsel or even knew of the ADR specialist role. Unfortunately the author recognized the difficulty many of my surgeon colleagues experienced in the role of compassionate provider. This required a split personality and some element of acting from many of these providers. The surgeon who, because of time constraints, higher litigation exposure, demanding personality typology (or disorder in my case), are probably the least sensitive of all providers to the social and psychological nuances that frame these difficult conversations. Not that surgeons are misguided, afraid or purposely reticent, but on the contrary, the problem is that delivering bad news is a routine part of most surgeon's job and many become desensitized to its impact on the patient and family. Considering the information and context for these delicate conversations, as a medical ADR consultant, the author always concentrated on the surgeons' approach and ability to interact with the family, and less about writing a specific script for the doctor to deliver.

As a brief corollary story, when I was a faculty member during my medical career, I interviewed applicants yearly for the neurosurgery residency. These young people all had impressive CVs and dedicated academic credentials or they would not have made the interview process. I posed the following scenario to every applicant, requesting they not share with their competitor, lest the position may be taken by that competitor who had time to consider their response to the following: 'you doctor have just had your patient die during surgery. This was a possibility discussed with patient and family before the case, but quite unexpected. Come out of the OR and tell me this news. Then, ask for the families authorization to donate the organs.' Stressful, right! Usually the applicant assumed a third position observer role, describing how 'they would do this' but I quickly interrupted them and reestablished the challenge. 'No, I am the father of the patient that just died. Talk to me.' The reader can ponder how they would respond, but until these difficult conversations become real, the provider cannot truly know how they will react to these situations.

It did take quite some time to establish trust with my colleagues, stepping away from my administrator or surgeon's role, and assuming the conflict management mantle. A certain level of calculus-based trust is necessary when guaranteeing I would remain impartial during disputes and hold information confidential. My colleagues and staff knew me as a surgeon who performed authoritative administrative roles as prior chairman of surgery and member of the credentialing and peer review quality assurance committees.

Sometimes I was quite averse to practitioners as I assumed the responsibility of these administrative positions. Therefore, this author suggests that any healthcare provider pursuing further education to assume the position of ADR medical specialist within their own institutions, takes the necessary time to secure relationships and be open and forthcoming about your transitional role to ADR advocate. Investigate and keep confidential the culture and personalities of as many of the medical staffers as you might access. Only with self-disclosure and professionalism will you develop the necessary credibility to achieve the trust and respect required to effectively manage dispute resolution, negotiation and mediation, when adversarial confrontations between staff members occur and patient-provider conflicts arise.

An excellent early step is to provide soundbite information on negotiation tactics focusing on collaborative interests. Offer insight, applying dispute resolution theory when dealing with colleagues in your organization. Interjecting a few thoughts and suggestions, although not primarily a mediator's job, supports a coaching and facilitator role that is enthusiastically received by staff and providers. The full deployment of the conflict resolution professional talent will be achieved using these micro victories, establishing oneself as the "go-to" person when arguments develop.

The curb side suggestions and brief interactions help establish that third-party authority as a consultant. In addition, at the highest level of disputes, such as formal mediation or arbitration, one can pierce that glass ceiling with expertise in healthcare by asserting the critical need for balanced information processing and communications during negotiations between disputants. Currently these professional positions are barren of medical practitioners. Sophisticated medical experience coupled with procedural legal understanding is the next evolution for a fair dispute resolution systems. Studies confirm that during private litigation using a panel with at least one arbitrator having subject matter expertise, such as a healthcare provider, results in greater stakeholder satisfaction and perception that the resolution was fair and impartial.

As a third-party neutral and subject matter expert, the healthcare ADR provides fresh insight into how an outsider, such as a jury, would view aspects of the dispute when paid experts are advocating for opposite conclusions. The role of subject matter expert supports credible suggestions regarding negotiation ranges and settlements and provides justification for plaintiffs, healthcare providers and insurance company representatives to utilize alternative dispute resolution to conclude the claim. Early mediation should be advocated to employ the discussed interest-based techniques before late stage evaluative mediation rules the exchange.

The healthcare ADR interviews as a clinician would, discusses positions relevant to a medical perspective unrestricted by discovery rules of alleged facts or evidence supporting only a legal argument. Once again, the disadvantages of evaluative mediation is the devaluation of emotional and psychological catharsis found in the deeper psychoanalytical approaches to conflict resolution. It is highly improbable that a monetary settlement will heal the wounds of distrust and malevolence found in late stage judicially-ordered evaluative exchange. To truly resolve a dispute, both plaintiff and defendant must process and understand each other's position, forgiving with empathy and peace building in mind. This medical ADR professional finds this very challenging when the focus is on a distributed demand encouraged by representative lawyers, limited by the desire for economic gain.

Another frequent request for a medical ADR services is to manage a disruptive healthcare provider's behavior. These requests come from administration, medical boards and from peer communication and often involve high conflict personality types that border on narcissism and egomania. This often requires an intervention that circumvents the traditional healthcare system hierarchy. Although these are often my most challenging cases, by applying strong negotiation skills using the jujitsu approach previously discussed, with a clear explanation of likely ramifications the provider can expect by continuing this behavior, for the most part, I have been able to teach these providers to alternatively express their desires and interests in a less combative manner.

Most providers, by their nature, assume the default positions of responsibility and behave in a command and control method of care delivery. All too often this author as the ADR specialist, consulting in very dysfunctional hospital systems, discovers these organizations never approach healthcare as "we are responsible" for the good and the bad. They are embroiled in the blame game, accusing providers with: 'doctor this is your patient and any problems are your problems.' As a result, these providers treat hospitals and their staff as a custodial way-stations to accomplish a task. Whether a provider is a superior care deliverer or not, they will always demand that the hospital function perfectly, efficiently, and without error. Demanding providers often require the hospital and clinic to accommodate to his/her schedule while providing that custodial care, assuming the patient will be delivered safely at the discharge date. Therein lies the paradox, neither the provider nor the medical staff are omnipotent or perfect. Neither are autonomous. The litany of twists and turns in medical care provided to each patient whose physiology probably will not respect a bell-shaped treatment curve, perfectly exemplifies management at the edge of chaos.

Every patient is a complex adaptation of scientific systems and pathophysiology. Unless providers and hospital staff are synchronized in communication and work harmoniously to deliver an integrative solution, their common goals and interests of quality and safety objectives will never be accomplished. Healthcare systems are in desperate need of proactive education and expedient intervention with conflict management systems to avoid the resultant bilateral anger, resentment, and legal entanglement occurring when treatment complications occur. Hospital systems or providers should not blame each other following adverse events. Although high profile conflicts in a medical organization center around adverse events and bad outcomes, the majority of disputes occur between the various healthcare providers. These require far more attention and if investigated and managed, will endear the ADR specialist's role within the institution.

Finally, as a neurosurgeon, I can unequivocally testify to the disruption, demoralization and dehumanization that occurs when the practitioner faces administrative and tort accusations. Often an unfortunate outcome or misjudgment by a provider explodes into a process of recrimination and even criminalization, as if the underlying act were a calculated intrusion designed to cause intentional harm to the very patient the provider is sworn to serve. The second victim experience is real and responsible for depression, burn out and in its extreme, provider suicide. In addition, the constant competition, one-upmanship and power struggles within healthcare systems can overwhelm any provider.

The ADR advocate must identify and aggressively manage all of these issues. This medical ADR professional objectively assess the medical consequences of perceived errors, investigates and pursues interpersonal conflicts and constructs systems to negotiate solutions and defuse adversaries. The ADR serves as the facilitating and mediating bridge, encouraging empathetic understanding and necessary communication, through impartial but experienced eyes.

Once trusted within the organization, the ADR specialist establishes programs and teaches medical staff to develop and subsequently intervene with their own conflict management skills. This author enjoys a fulfilling and exceptionally rewarding advisory management position supporting ADR intervention and qualitative initiatives designed to ensure excellence in care delivery within medical organizations.

The author's common experience when working with providers with limited ADR knowledge understands, and is not surprised, that the term mediation creates a visceral repulsion in medical staff. Mediation is synonymous with the litigation process. Most healthcare providers with any experience in litigation were challenged as to their judgment and the quality of their medical practice. Thus, there are very few neurons between 'medical malpractice lawsuit' and mediation experience. In fact, prior to the authors interest and subsequent education in the ADR discipline, I also understood mediation as a pre-trial requirement. At mediation the provider is in an alien environment and feels powerless. Lawyers in charge demand a negotiated solution, where the provider is coerced to capitulate to a settlement, allowing the insurance adjusters to try and drive down the value of a medical malpractice claim. Even with frivolous claims the mantra is "get the case settled," despite great defenses against the claim.

The pessimist view is that litigation is nothing more than an economic machine controlled by and for the exclusive benefit of lawyers. These processes are not elective and entrap providers whose only hope for justice maybe an impartial judge willing to separate what is right from wrong. Unfortunately, having participated in the evaluative mediation process as an expert, a defendant and as a consultant, the author can attest that these experiences are polar opposite to the interest-based negotiation advocated by ADR professionals. Traditional pre-trial mediation attempts to convince both parties that the trial process, regardless of strength in argument, is too risky and unpredictable. From this limited perspective, the label of mediator is a scarlet letter lost in the healthcare organization.

To that end, as a consultant the author's official title is: *Conflict Engagement Specialist.* The job requires an experienced practitioner inquisitive and engaging, attempting to unseal the vault of stoic healthcare professional's personalities. As medical providers we are hell bent to convince the world we are right, quickly assume a dispositional and defensive posture when challenged, and often respond emotionally to perceived threats challenging our authority. A seasoned medical ADR's goal is to reframe their colleagues perspective and embrace opportunities to create and participate in a collaborative and strategic healthcare system supported by a conflict management providing dispute resolution.

APPENDIX ONE

The author is a principal at Provider Resolutions, LLP, located at https://www.provider-resolutions.com. Here is an example of a successful communication following an introductory letter where a large private medical insurance carrier requested we specifically describe our procedures as ADR specialists before hiring our firm:

Provider Resolutions, LLP shall prepare the template and orchestrate the structural paradigm by which our experts will facilitate stakeholder communication, pre-meeting caucus, intra-meeting group interaction and post meeting negotiations and follow through. Concentration on common goals, topic discussions, contract negotiations, contract execution and the system tracking function necessary to ensure both the ACO and +++(national third party payor) comply with the contract specifications, including reporting, error tracking and relationship management. Importantly, a grievance process will be agreed upon in which both parties will attend to the issues within a preset time frame, investigating resolution and if required, contacting Provider Resolution specialists as the intermediary to mediate for dispute resolution.

This proposed model identifies and invites key stakeholders and decision makers who must participate in this congress to accomplish the contractual tasks required to provide defined medical services and obtain reimbursement for those services. Both groups are required to submit a brief description of their key personnel necessary to accomplish this task. Those key persons are requested to submit a letter of intent to negotiate in good faith, participate actively in the discussion leading to an acceptable contract and provide a goal statement for public consumption as a pre-meeting introduction of whom they are as participating members of this contracting convention. Our model as facilitators is to explore 'individual stakeholder perceptions and look at common goals.' As facilitators our mission requires a formulation of a new reality in which both sides arrive at multiple collaborative agreements and the facilitator then supports the collective new definition of the relationship between parties as 'the collective agreements.' This new socially created knowledge base is the definition of the new relationship, accepting the terms of a negotiated agreement as truth. We intend to utilize these 'social learning models' for consensus building when two or more parties claim a position based upon their desired dispositional perspective.

The discourse objective for the group negotiation is critical to helping multiple perspectives converge on shared knowledge. The accumulation of negotiated shared knowledge results in the establishment of an accepted group perspective.

Thank you,

Michael Schneider, MD MS-ADR,

Principal Provider Resolutions, LLP

www.provider-resolutions.com

APPENDIX TWO

The ombudsman role: Conversations with patients and families following adverse outcomes:

Apology:

I'm so very sorry this has happened to you ...

We are terribly sorry that these actions caused this kind of pain and worry.

I'm so very sorry for your loss (or recent experience) and I'm here to assist in any way I can.

Empathetic Statements

You have every right to be upset. This is so different from what we wanted to happen.

The whole team is heartbroken that ...

We are devastated by what has happened here

You must feel the weight of the world on your shoulders.

You must be angry ... frustrated ... outraged by what has occurred here ...

I can see you are really upset ... devastated ... angry

This is just shocking ...

Wanting to understand our patients and families:

I am here to listen (or assist) you. Is this a good time to talk?

If you would like to tell me what is going on, I would like to hear what happened.

Tell me what it is you know ... (way to understand the person's perception)

This is a devastating situation, what is on your mind ... what are your concerns and needs right now?

How can I be helpful?

Tell me what I need to know.

Continuing the Conversation & Gaining More Understanding:

We (I) know this must be so difficult for you, if you need a break at any time, we understand ... We (I) appreciate you letting us know your needs.

Help me understand ... (then reframe what you heard) ..... did I leave anything out?

Is there anything else we can do for your family right now? We have some support here. What do you need that would be helpful?

Planning for next steps:

When I talk about successfully addressing your concerns, what does it look like to you?

Have I heard all your concerns? Have I covered all your concerns?

Here is what I all/ able to do ...

We are already taking steps to see that this will not happen to someone else.

We don't know and understand what happened yet and we want to find out as soon as possible.

Thank you for your time and honesty. Here is what I am going to do.

If your family or relatives come to the hospital, ask them to call this number and myself/or one of my staff will speak to them.

I want to tell you what happened to the best of my ability and discuss what we are proposing to do next in discussion with you.

I want to show you that we are doing everything we can to care for you and support you. I am wanting to review with you and your family what we know and how we are proceeding.

Care Team:

Each clinician takes his/her responsibility very seriously. There will be a great deal of self-analysis over how this could have happened. Would it help if I explained why this diagnosis can be so difficult to make early on?

We take care of patients as a team, and it would be unfair to hold an individual fully responsible for something that others might also have been able to help catch.

We often have to wait for a disease to show itself more fully before we can reliably detect and treat it.

We know it can be confusing when we appear to change our explanation and yet, as more facts became available to us, we realized that our initial impressions of what had likely happened were incorrect.

Would it help if I explained the medical situation as it looked to me at that point? I know that it may be harder to trust us now that we have acknowledged our error.

<u>Unknown causes</u>
We are conducting a thorough investigation right now and I will personally call you immediately when I have any information to share with you.
We don't know why/how/where/when this happened. We ask for your patience while we do all that we can to find out.
We might not ever fully know how this heart-breaking event occurred.

APPENDIX THREE

EXAMPLES OF MEDIATED CONFLICT RESOLUTION IN THE
HEALTHCARE SETTING. REFERENCING ACADEMIA AND
RESOLVING THE DISPUTES.

A. **The Group practice breaking up.**

An established group with aging senior and original partners is
in conflict with the younger members, and the fractured future
competitors will weaken their strength in the market place. The
practice really has two parties fundamentally in conflict, the
original practice owners and the other group of physicians
seeking autonomy and recognition. At the core of the conflict
are values issues related to the identity of the practice and the
identity of the individual. The founding members of this
practice and the practices success are likely the alter ego of this
person, thus any compromise to his way of doing business will
be an insult to his core identity-based recognition. The
opponents view of course is their need for self-determination,
both personally and professionally and to escape totalitarian
rule. The current model of this group is not sustainable and if
the group breaks up, the animosity and personal and
professional attacks will affect the entire medical community.

1. The Wheel of conflict, created by Bernie Mayer, PhD
   and Chris Moore, PhD has key elements allowing the
   conflict professional to understand and organize the

231

needs and interests of the individuals in a dispute while moving through the different stages of conflict interaction, while considering the cognitive, emotional and behavioral aspects that impact attempts at conflict resolution.

- These are: the structure of the relationship between parties or structure of interaction that defines their communication; the emotional influence on both rational and irrational behaviors and decisions of all parties in how they perceive and react to the conflict experience; the historical interaction with both positive and negative experiences between the parties; the functional communication between opponents, from both verbal and nonverbal interaction; the relative value of not only the potential outcome from a resolution to the conflict but the significance of the conflict itself and the impact it has on the opponents self-identity and needs.

2. Application of a Complexity theory perspective to intervention requires a disruptive perspective. The traditional practice management hierarchy in this group is stifling and dictates roles and procedures, expecting every person to adapt to the rigidity of the structure.

- The organization discounts the autonomy of individual agents and how they will act and react within the structure and how co-workers function within the structure, setting up exponential opportunities for conflict. Complexity theory requires us to look at the group through the lens of a complex adaptive system, realizing that the relationships will govern the implementation of the structure and not the other way around.

- Therefore, integrating Group dynamic theory into the complex adaptive system, we see the need for broad strokes of "good enough" vision of the future within this group, defining general concepts and simplifying them to core needs and interests of each of the parties. There will be competition for relevance in those conversations, but complex adaptive systems encourage the tension and harnessed its energy to respectful communication that should lead to discovery of ideas and opportunities that only the group dynamic interaction would have discovered.

3. In the back ground are the murmurs of unexpressed ideas, disgruntled interpretations of past interaction and current disaffected complaints communicated through the "shadow system" of chatter and information flow.

   - This system and these communications reflect raw and unfiltered feelings and should be revealed and explored, as it will reflect how the group will integrate changes believed to be positive and functional.

   - Commitment by all parties is critical to the ultimate mission, so discovering the essence of thoughts that lie at the fringes, modify ideas and morph opportunities into reality, when addressing changes and modifications of the status quo.

   - Changes should be introduced in small increments, so as not to be trampled by the overwhelming behemoth that each group member sees as their future path. The suggestion of global change without a method of discovery will prove disastrous for this group's future.

4. The focus of the ADR professional's facilitation should be to provide structure to the elements of the conflict,

understanding the needs and interest-based issues as simply job security, economic and professional decision autonomy, all within the group mission of mutual success through business collaboration.

- This requires creation of a functional democratic mechanism that gives each partner a voice. All this must be accomplished by demonstrating the problems of the current hierarchy to the anyone wielding more 'power over' instead of 'power with', and will only be successful if the originating partner truly has interests beyond his own ego and pocket book.

- The ADR consultant will analyze the dysfunctional group and create a diagram showing the pathophysiology of this group – totalitarian rule, fragmented communication resulting in distrust and also outline the risks going forward under current doctrine that created this divided practice.

- The ADR spends time on values of a democracy and what each of those values means to each stakeholder, and lastly explores the history of the group to see if democracy was considered in the past, and what was the result. The ADR professional is the truth seeker here and demonstrating that to everyone involved should meet the ADR professional's core needs.

5. The ultimate negotiations should occur when senior partners understand the next generation has identical values to themselves that must be fulfilled. The value proposition aligns mutual interests and underscores the threat of a mirrored competitive practice with younger competitors should the practice divide.

   - In addition, group identity must respect individual autonomy, proportional work effort and rules of reimbursement for each provider. The management challenges to running the practice becomes the common ground for negotiations.

6. The ADR separates the people from the problem (Fisher & Ury), where the people are the patients and the problem is the money generated from the work. A method of fair revenue reimbursement for personnel based upon work effort and a shared pool, or slush fund, added to the productivity revenue structure is agreed upon.

- Democratic decisions regarding the administrative side of the practice are then constructed easily and efficiently managed by consensus opinion.

B. **The Charge Nurse conflict. Authority vs Respect.**

1. Understanding the dimensions of interpersonal conflict as it causes dysfunctional relationships in the work place is a critical human resource function required of the ADR professional. As we can see from this scenario, work relationships between employees and management influence the peace, civility and functionality of the work environment. To maintain professionalism and continue to focus on patient care, all employees must experience shared mutual respect. In this conflict we can look at structure, referring to the dynamics of the participant's authority and power-over or power-with between the charge nurse and the staff nurse.

2. When one party feels threatened, and in this case when the charge nurse and staff nurse fail to respect one another, this ensures a communication void that deepens the conflict.

- Not uncommonly, the person with less authority such as the staff nurse, might rely on intimidation to "control" the relationship with the charge nurse, depleting the perception of power-over by negating the charge nurse's authority.

- Emotional dispositional positions govern this relationship with fear and anger clouding the functional integrative relationship needed for both parties to complete their professional tasks.

3. Both nurses perceive they are under attack by their opponent. Clearly the relationship does not hold value for either nurse, even if the work does.

   - Animosity is freely expressed as the staff nurse feels the charge nurse is unkind and critically reviews her work practice. The charge nurse feels vulnerable and has concerns about her responsibility to ensure quality patient care.

   - Determining the historical interaction between these two rivals allows an ADR professional to determine the depth of past offenses and look for opportunities to find common ground through appreciative inquiry.

4. If the etiology of this conflict is truly related to alternative care delivery views, that opposition should be explored by an ADR professional to understand how each person's values regarding their care delivery result in negative interpersonal relationship full of venom and acrimony.

    - Fundamentally, humans desire respect and recognition of their efforts and importance from their social group, including the work place. This is a core value proposition common in all members of the healthcare team.

5. Leadership and organizational principles supporting the complexity of these relationships concentrates on effective communication to lead conflict through to "uncover and work with paradox and tension."

    - According to Mayer, "values are the beliefs we have about what is important, what distinguishes right from wrong and good from evil, and what principles should govern how we live our lives". Recognizing when core values are opposed or belittled, plays an important role in conflict resolution and implicit in effective communication between these two dispositional parties.

6. An ADR professional should bring both nurses into a safe conflict support zone for communication and intervention.

   - Once conversation is established and core needs addressed, the goal for mutual understand and appreciation must be reached for both parties to return to the work environment.
   - The ADR frames the work place requiring a peaceful, efficient and safe location for staff and patients.
   - The ADR professional thus injects the system values on the parties as a frame to influence a collaborative work project designed to repair this relationship.

7. Although medicine is governed by hierarchy, innovation in patient care delivery for efficiency and collegiality might present significant opportunities where these two nurses could work together in a collegial fashion, not as boss and subordinate, but equal as it relates to an objective outcome of quality health initiatives.

- Working together under the concept of complexity science will stimulate clumping of ideas and interaction with colleagues other than the two in conflict.

- The working peer group must support the new collaborative relationship. The shadow system, gossip and rumor mill so prevalent in the hospital work place can be used to the ADR professional's advantage.

- A repaired relationship between these two adversaries will quickly spread through the informal shadow information system giving both traction and consent to support the communication and respect obviated by the repaired relationship. How these two nurses subsequently interact will have a significant impact on the entire floor/ward that is not predictable, but hopefully beneficially influential. This single event with its ripple and interactive influence is the fundamental concept behind complex adaptive systems.

- By repairing this relationship, the ADR professional might create phenomenon throughout the group that stimulates a healthier and more productive work environment for all employees.

C. **The hierarchical dilemma infused with burnout and impatience.**

1. The hospital administrator calls in an ADR consultant because staff satisfaction is demoralized, and patient complaints are at a fever pitch. The incidence of errors in medication delivery are increasing and the hospital just lost an ugly medical malpractice lawsuit and was thrashed by the local paper.

   - The organization suffers from clinical and personnel miscommunication that has reached a critical level and is threatening patient safety. Like most hospitals, they are inhibited by the hierarchical nature and command and control behavior of senior highly educated members of the healthcare team.

   - There is an inverse relationship between time in contact with the patient and their family, and the level of education.

     - The physician may spend 15-20 minutes a day at the bedside when managing a patient however but the young nursing staff, from CNA to new nurses, have the most contact and are in a position to observe and evaluate critical changes in patient's status.

2. The senior nurses are shorthanded and relegated to passing out meds, changing IV solutions and performing the record documentation on a large number of patients.

3. The various members of the team are not comfortable expressing concerns over patient care because of draconian and abusive supervision.

   - Limited communication occurs because staff feels that intimidation and harsh verbal dismissals often occur when a more senior person believes the junior person should have knowledge that would answer the juniors' concerns. Important questions are trivialized. The senior's answers are often trite, curt and designed to embarrass the junior person to prevent a similar "stupid" question from occurring again.

   - The different medical team members have poor professional relationship that are dispositional, disrespectful and angry, resulting in failure to communicate important care issue. This vicious circle results in mistakes through the hospital. When they occur, parties begin to blame each other, and the relationships break down further. Interactions are acrimonious, guarded and precarious.

4. The shadow communication network spreads gossip and negative attributions about the providers, nurses and techs throughout the healthcare system. A conflict between two parties quickly recruits many more staff members, creating the deleterious effect on staff morale and future patient care.

   - The noxious environment spreads through discourteous and limited professional exchange that further restrict collaborative team work.
   - The patients are suffering inferior care and recognize themselves as victims, condemning the facility and provider reputations with bad social media posts and media attacks.

5. The ADR professional has many challenges here and recruits additional experienced dispute resolution specialists to tackle this project and effect meaningful system change.

- Fundamentally, every level of healthcare providers should be required to complete training in conflict recognition, integrative and collaborative group theory, and team building with open communication training to support the global safe healthcare mission.

- The organization can introduce a stepwise approach that embraces the core concepts of conflict resolution by establishing a systematic study to identify the various aspects of conflict in this system, the stress points causing conflict, and establish access points to a long-term independent ADR professional, available to quickly defuse disputes and improve communication within the hospital.

6. An ombudsman and an ADR professional must be hired and formally identified in the system. These professionals engage in intense 'facetime' at every level of provider in this system. Their active listening and supportive approach triggers their acceptance as compassionate neutrals available to assist patients, their families and the medical staff. As an institutional asset,

the ADR office will be prominently featured in the staff, provider and patient information packets.

- The imperative demonstrates the administrations dedication to the medical staff, reiterating their work philosophy must quell disputes and focus on a patient centered mission.
- The ADR office mandate is responsive through reflective understanding of events.
- The ADR professional institutes conflict prevention techniques and develops multiple points of entry for patients and staff to access the ADR service. These include office hours, call in, email, text and anonymous complaint containers.
- All staff acknowledge there is no retribution for voicing a complaint and every concern will be addressed. Open and honest communication is the most effective strategy toward mitigating damages to trust and respect between team members.

7. The ADR office works closely with human resources, identifying issues that rise above an ADR management issue, such as violence in the work place, or issues that require administrative intervention because of dangerous behavior.

- The ADR person ethically understands these issues must be discussed with proper authorities within the organization before attempting any intervention. Work place harassment may be identified by the ADR office discovery and despite rules of confidentiality, the civil and criminal implications of adverse actions demand legal counsel available through the HR office.

8. Employment and credentialing within the institution requires continuing education and participation in an internal communications ADR driven morbidity and mortality conference on a quarterly basis.

9. The ADR office and specifically the ombudsman works closely with healthcare providers on empathic apologies, mitigating economic damages in para litigious negotiations after an adverse event.
   - Errors management requires coordination with administration and legal counsel.
   - Medical and nursing staff policies are matured and streamlined to evaluate and act upon mistakes that fall below the standard of care.

10. Through continuous education in ADR techniques, extenders whose primary work remains in healthcare then champion the ADR techniques throughout the hospital and clinics, with operational aspects of facilitation available to assist in this systematic deployment of conflict management practices.

- The ADR office is responsible for continuous training and updating medical staff to remain relevant and responsive.

D. A truly toxic and hostile work environment.

A letter sent to www.Provider-Resolutions.com requesting our intervention:

Dear Dr Schneider,

Our organization is suffering from the cancerous wrath of interpersonal conflict, back biting and unregulated angry discrimination that threatens our human resource infrastructure and compromises our ability to deliver superior safe patient care. Our mission statement is under attack and we must change the culture of organization, implementing several critical pathways to stem this non-physical work place violence. The anger and negative attitudes present impediments to the organizations cohesive growth and the partnership we represent in shepherding the infirmed and their families through their healthcare crisis. We are collaterally victimizing the patient and their families as they look to us for professional medical care and compassionate understanding during their crisis. Instead we act in a self-serving and destructive manner when we fail to institute rules that demand everyone on our staff will respect and create a harmonized work environment that is supportive, respectful, mindful and professional to their co-workers. We recently had a screaming match between two doctors in front of the nurses' station with family and patients left aghast. This once again exemplifies the direct distain and personality combat bringing this issue again to the forefront of much needed management intervention to quickly deal with these quality improvement threats. Thank you, Susan........ Board Member at 275 bed hospital on the East coast.

1. A perspective of the impact of this hostile work environment has on all stake holders references Maxfield's work with the AORN and AACN on "The silent treatment." This 2010 study of 6500 nurses and nurse managers discussed the impact of compromised communication for any reason in the healthcare work environment.

   - The study demonstrated that hostility between personnel creates this miscommunication and prevents sharing critical patient data. As Maxfield illustrates when healthcare professionals' fail to raise concerns when risks are identified due to acrimonious interchange with co-workers, this undermines the effectiveness of patient care safety tools resulting in dangerous shortcuts, incompetence and disrespect between team members and toward patients.

- Personnel hostility is profoundly discourteous, affecting each participant and the failure to communicate beeches provider's ethical responsibilities. In addition, the tension created through unresolved interpersonal conflicts is a form of lateral bullying and workplace violence. This issue is raised in several respectable journals and on-line forums.

  - Gerardi addresses this as a critical breaking point in the hospital work place. She describes the use of mediation techniques to identify conflict early and develop a plan to resolve the dispute by "listening, reframing the concerns raised, identifying commonalities and clearly defining decisions".

  - The author supports her position that 'effective conflict management in the clinical setting include, being present in the moment, listening for understanding, mutuality, openness, and reflection.'

2. Provider Resolutions, LLP has at our disposal, several experienced dispute resolution specialist including the author who identified people within the organization either trained or expressing a desire to be trained in conflict management techniques.

    - The senior administration identified establishing a conflict resolution platform as critical to the hospitals mission.

        - As Maxfield solutions suggest '... when it comes to creating healthy work environments that ensure optimal quality of care, individual skills and personal motivation won't be enough to reduce harm and save lives unless speaking up is also supported by the social and structural elements within the organization. Changing entrenched behavior in healthcare organizations will require a multifaceted approach that leaders can follow to improve people's ability to hold crucial conversations.'

- Guidelines implemented must be memorialized and employees alongside medical staff must sign contracts committing to resolutions agreed upon within the organization. The institutional commitment is critical at every level and mandates required participation in conflict engagement interviews, mediations, coaching and counseling when appropriate.

3. Of the broad conflict management system we recommended, one section specifically addressed work place hostility.

   - The doctrine we created and subsequently enacted included: multiple pathways to identify and access the system of conflict management for providers and employees; an outline for reporting abuse stressing a safe and confidential communication platform where personnel need not worry about subsequent discrimination, retaliation, or termination; the process the hospital will follow to address reported behavior and remedy the issue; the method of investigation of accusations and corrective education when abuse has occurred; and the follow up communication plans for the person reporting the issue.

4. Prior to enacting this system, the author stood before the entire hospital staff and providers, read the letter soliciting our assistance (redacting the author) and delivered this imperative: "We have excellent opportunities to improve our healthcare delivery and minimize errors and omissions by supporting conflict management in healthcare. First, we must present a unified and cohesive action plan to all of you and allow you time to embrace the concepts and add to the identification process and ideas for resolution of these conflicts as you are all key stakeholders in this process. I promise that implementing a conflict identification and resolution system will protect your patients while improving the atmosphere in your work environment. I am confident your professional and personal lives will be enriched if you commit to this process. I believe the JCHO mandate of 2009 demands we pay attention to these issues and that that the interpersonal conflict between staff locked in angry avoidance exemplifies the difficulty your organization has with poor

communication. This is a very real and present danger to your patients and your psychological well-being. We cannot tolerate this behavior and provide a safe, effective, and compassionate work environment. I implore the administrative governing body to adopt techniques of conflict management into the professional training of every staff member and employee and make the training and surveillance of your organization in dispute management a critical priority to your survival. The cost of lost man power hours and staff turn-over is crippling your organization and the patients know it."

- We then followed up with a written summary to all personnel, soliciting buy in from the staff. The opportunities inherent in a conflict management system include: recognition of conflict as an indicator to allow early identification of problems, promotion of a proactive response to problems and conflict, encouragement of a culture of mutual respect, open communication, problem solving during inquiry or intervention relating to conflict, and a means of working towards potential resolution.

- The tenants of our management system will emphasize a willingness to acknowledge existence of conflict; open communication between all team members; dealing with conflict within an environment of mutual respect; acceptance and tolerance of different perspectives through the process; commitment to fundamental fairness; educating all staff about conflict management in healthcare; continually reflecting on and modifying our policies and procedures with input from every employee and provider and then holding administration, providers and staff accountable to use the conflict management process.

5. Although this broken system required months to implement the platform and there was substantial pain following the termination of some very high conflict individuals, including threatened de-credentialing and medical board action against two very toxic physicians, the result was worth the struggle.

   ▪ The author returned for one week every six months for two years back to this organization tuning up the ADR communication and delivery agenda and engaging both staff and providers to confirm the good health of the dispute resolution platform.

APPENDIX FOUR

Reader Case challenges

Common Scenarios where the medical ADR uses an interest-based style of conflict management to work on resolution. The reader is tasked with analysis and reframing options in each conflict situation. Utilize the exchange interest-based mediation approach and as a provider, temper the default evaluative bias tempting you to suggest solutions before active listening to each party. Identify key stakeholders, address the conflict and recommend you action plan. How will you question and reframe emotional professionals? How will you avoid advocating for one side? How will you neutralize power differentials?

The reader is referenced to read and contribute to the blog at www.provider-resolutions.com/healthcare-conlfict-scenerios

The reader can collaborate with interested medical ADR professionals, incorporating innovative ideas into your own practice by contributing your unique perspective in conflict resolution.

Cases:

1. The provider arrives on the floor to find that her orders were not carried out to the letter and explodes in a tirade in front of the patient and their family.

2. There is a fundamental disagree on relevance of information regarding care management in this case. Nursing believes certain issues are relevant, but the physician disregards the concerns without any specific explanation. Animosity develops between nursing staff and the physician.

3. There are multiple physicians not integrating care in an ICU patient. At various times the physician's frustration is vented onto the nurse treating the patient who becomes angered and confused as to what is appropriate care and annoyed over the derogatory comments about other physicians with whom she maintains a respectful professional relationship. This miscommunication threatens quality of care.

4. Two nurses disagreeing over the timing, documentation and relevance of the information about a common patient such as change in shift and the derogatory conversations that occur from both sides afterward with other staff members –

   i. The shadow system reports back to the original nurses about these comments. Dysfunctional relationships develop in which their sniping and bad-mouthing fosters inappropriate criticism.

5. Patient/family don't like the way the nurse/the therapist is treating them and complains to their Nurse Practitioner, making accusations about quality, trying to enlist the NP to their bias, as they perceive the NP will condemn the nurse/therapist.

   i. There is an element of dark satisfaction on the part of the patient when they create conflict and use the senior person in the traditional hierarchy as their advocate/ surrogate to criticize someone perceived as lower on the hierarchical chain.

ii. How does this impact long term distrust between care givers? Does the provider recognize the patients manipulative behavior?

iii. Hint - the mediator desires to repair that relationship between patient and all care givers and not just embarrass the patient, creating a 'loser' in this scenario.

1. When the mediator represents a common value theme within the organization, she reframes the conflict generated by the patient confirming that everyone is integral to the healthcare team. The value and trust that each type of between providers must also be revealed and maintained.

2. The ADR addresses all parties concerns and the process of resolution will not be punitive.

6. Demanding providers who complain about administrative processes, quality of other department's care, demands in the operating room, and believes the loud squeaky wheel will reward their demands.

    i. The mediator is correct when they influence this provider to create and enact solutions to their complaints.

7. ERROR management – communication, disclosure, what the patient and family wants – what happens when this is ignored, and a plaintiff's attorney begins to coach the adversarial patient.

    i. How should the ADR address medical mistakes?

8. Dispute over modification of a long-standing care plan policy or procedure.

    i. Hint – who are the stakeholders? Who can make the decisions? How are changes communicated throughout the system?

9. Anger and hostility that fracture relationships when providers disagree on care management decisions.

    i. Hint – attribution errors? Appreciative inquiry to repair a relationship? Valuation of current dispute over long term collaborative positions?

10. A provider is reported by an anonymous communication to the ADR office as possibly being impaired. Alcohol is detectable on the provider's breathe. What steps does the ADR take to intervene for patient safety?

11. Conflict between two radiology technicians from an outside dispute is carried over to hostile behavior in the outpatient clinic. The disruptive behavior affect several other people in the outpatient work environment.

12. Several younger nurses are posting Facebook comments that target one older nurse they have a tense and acrimonious relationship with.

      i. How can the ADR influence behavior outside of the workplace? Does the ADR have the right or authority to do so?

          1. Hint – reframe your approach and resist an initial punitive approach to the young nurses. Engaging all nurses with the evidence at hand, exploring the foundations of the conflict, the emotional cost of the attack, etc.

13. Surgeons are complaining that the O.R. staff are all visiting techs who are not qualified to participate in their cases. This has caused escalating anger and dysfunctional relationship between the operating room nurse manager, several surgeons and the few nurses that are full time staff. Initial inquiry discovers a much larger problem set with complaints including timing, turn over and even PACU quality of care initiatives.

      i. Who are the stakeholders and how will the ADR bring the large group of surgeons together with administration? Is it necessary to have all of the surgeons at every meeting?

14. The provider is a significant contributor to the hospitals bottom line and her patients love her but nursing staff, technicians and even ward clerks find the provider demanding, aloof and discourteous. The administration does not want to upset the provider because of their financial contribution and the provider's public image is quite important to the hospital's board members.

   i. Hint – conflict arises when two parties identify an issue and take positions against each other. Who are the conflicted parties here? Can the ADR make an ally with this provider and how would that influence the provider's perception of themselves seen through the eyes of her work colleagues?

The interested reader may seek further insight into conflict engagement and dispute resolution by accessing a two hour animated video lecture series, including several entertaining health care conflict scenarios and their management at:

https://www.udemy.com/conflict-engagement-for-the-healthcare-provider/learn/v4/overview

Enter discount code: CONFLICT

Thank you. I hope this book improves your professional relationships and commitment to your own peace and contentment as a health care provider.

Bibliography

Angermeier, I, et al: (Mar/Apr 2009) The Impact of Participative Management Perceptions on Customer Service, Medical Errors, Burnout, and Turnover Intentions. J HC Mgmt 54(2).

Association for Conflict Resolution http://www.acrnet.org/

Balcerzak, G, Leonhardt, K Alternative Dispute Resolution in Healthcare. A Prescription for Increasing Disclosure and Improving Patient Safety. https://www.psqh.com/analysis/alternative-dispute-resolution-in-healthcare-a-prescription-for-increasing-disclosure-and-improving-patient-safety/

Berman, S. (2002, April). Reporting outcomes and other issues in patient safety: An interview with Albert Wu. Journal on Quality Improvement, 28, 197-204.

Blatt, R., Brown, M., & Lerner, J. (2001). Co-mediation: A success story at Chicago's Rush Medical Center. http://www.adrsystems.com/news/Co-Mediation.pdf

Bohn, D et al. (1991) Dialogue - a proposal. Infed.org. http://www.infed.org/archives/e-texts/bohm_dialogue.htm

Boothman, R. C. (March/April 2006). Apologies and a strong defense at the University of Michigan Health System. The Physician Executive, 7-10.

Brown, B Listening to shame. - http://www.ted.com/talks/brene_brown_listening_to_shame

Bryson, J. M., Crosby, B. C., & Stone, M. M. (2006). The Design and Implementation of Cross-Sector Collaborations: Propositions from the Literature. Public Administration Review, 66(S1), 44-55.

Camerer CF. (2003) Behavioral Game Theory: Experiments in Strategic Interaction. Princeton, NJ: Princeton University Press

Carlson, M. (1998). A model for improving a group. The Institute of Government.

CDA Collaborative Learning Projects
http://www.cdainc.com/cdawww/default.php

Chen, B., Graddy, E. (2005) . Inter- Organizational Collaborations for Public Service Delivery: A Framework of reconditions, Processes, and Perceived Outcomes. ARNOVA Conference, November 17 – 19, Washington, DC

Chen, P. (2009) Final Exam: A Surgeon's Reflection on Mortality. Random House Publishing NY.

Chong, P. S., & Benli, Ö S. (2005). Consensus in team decision making involving resource allocation. Management Decision, 43(9)

Cohen, J. R. (2004). Toward candor after medical error: The first apology law. Harvard Health Policy Review, 5.

Cooley, J. W. (2002). A dose of ADR for the health care industry. Dispute Resolution Journal.

Consensus Building Institute http://cbuilding.org/ and http://www.crinfo.org/

Dimock, H. (1985). How to observe your group. Centre for Human Resource Development, University of Guelph.

Dimock, H. and Kass, R., (2007). How to observe your group (4th edition). Captus Press; Concord, MA

Doyle, M. and Straus, D. (1993). How to make meetings work. Berkley Publishing Group.

Dressler, L. (2010). Standing in the fire: Leading high-heat meetings with clarity, calm, and courage. Berrett-Koehler Publishers; San Francisco, CA.

Dauer, E. (2004) Health Dispute and Risk Management http://www.preventivelawyer.org/main/default.asp?pid=health_dispute.htm

Endriss, U. Maudet, F., Toni. F. (2003) On optimal outcomes of negotiations over resources. In Proc. of AAMAS '03

Fisher, R., Ury, W., Patton, B. (2011) Getting to YES. Negotiating Agreements without Giving In. Penguin Group publishing, NY.

Forester, J. (2009) Dealing with differences: Dramas of mediating public disputes. Oxford University Press; New York, NY.

Foster, H., Schwartz, J., & DeRenzo, E. (2002, June 10). Reducing legal risk by practicing patient-centered medicine. Archives of Internal Medicine, 162

Gallagher, T. et al. (2006) Choosing your words carefully: How physicians would disclose harmful medical errors to patients. Archives of Internal Medicine 166.

Gallagher, T. et al (2003) Patients' and physicians' attitudes regarding the disclosure of medical errors. Journal of the American Medical Association, 289(8)

Gerardi, D. (2008) Lateral Violence and Bullying in the Workplace Using mediation techniques to manage conflict and create healthy work environments. AACN Clinical Issues: Advanced Practice in Acute & Critical Care, 15(2)

Gerardi, D. (2003) Conflict management training for health care professionals. http://www.mediate.com/articles/gerardi4.cfm

Gerding, E. et al (2000) Scientific approaches and techniques for negotiation: a game theoretic and artificial intelligence perspective. Technical report, SEN-R0005, CWI

Ghais, S. (2005). Extreme facilitation: Guiding groups through controversy and complexity. Jossey-Bass Publishers; San Francisco, CA.

Goodman, A. Basic Skills for the New Arbitrator, Second Edition. Solomon Publications.

Goodman, A. Basic Skills for the New Mediator, Second Edition. Solomon Publications.

Gray, B. (1989). Collaborating: Finding common ground for multiparty problems. Jossey-Bass Publishers; San Francisco, CA.

Greenwood, M.(2008) How to Mediate Like A Pro: 42 Rules for Mediating Disputes. iUniverse Press.
Guadagnino, C. (2004). Malpractice mediation poised to expand. Physician's News Digest.

Harvard Center for ADR – The Schwartz Center at http://www.theschwartzcenter.org/

Healthcare Professional Institute at https://healthprofessionalsinstitute.com/

Hickson, G. et al (1992). Factors that prompted families to file malpractice claims following perinatal injury. Journal of the American Medical Association. 287(10)

Houk, C. (2002, June). The internal neutral: Why doesn't your hospital have one? http://www.mediate.com/articles/houk.cfm

Houk, C, et al. (2008) Apology and Disclosure How a Medical Ombudsmen Can Help Bring a Policy to Life. http://www.psqh.com/mayjun08/apology.html

Hyman, C et al (2005): Interest-Based Mediation of Medical Malpractice Lawsuits: A Route to Improved Patient Safety? Journal of Health Politics. Policy and Law, Vol. 35,(5) Duke University Press

Isaacs, W. (1999). Dialogue and the art of thinking together: A pioneering approach to communicating in business and in life. Doubleday, Random House, Inc.; New York, NY

International Association of Facilitators. http://www.iaf-world.org/i4a/pages/index.cfm?pageid=1

Joint Commission Resources: 2011 Hospital Accreditation Standards. Oakbrook Terrace, Ill.: Joint Commission on Accreditation of Healthcare Organizations (JCAHO). (2007). Disclosing medical errors: A guide to an effective explanation and apology. Oak Park, IL: Joint Commission Resources.

Johnson, D. and Johnson, F. (2013). Joining together: Group theory and group skills. Pearson Education Inc.; NJ. (11th ed)

Klein, M., et al (2003) The Dynamics of Collaborative Design: Complex Systems and Negotiation Research. Understanding Complex Systems Complex Engineered Systems Current Engineering. Sage publication.

Klein, M: (2008) The Dynamics of Collaborative Design with Insights from Complex Systems and Negotiation System Sciences (HICSS)

Kaldjian, L (2007) Disclosing Medical Errors to Patients: Attitudes and Practices of Physicians and Trainees. J of General Internal Medicine(22)9.

Kaner, S., et al. (1996). Facilitator's guide to participatory decision-making. New Society Publishers; Gabriola Island, BC.

Kelsey, D. and Plumb, P. (1997). Great meetings! Hanson Park Press; Portland, ME.

Kahneman, D and Tversky, A.(2004) Conflict Resolution: A Cognitive Perspective in Preference, Belief, and Similarity Selected Writings of Amos Tversky. MIT Press.

Kohn, L., et al. (2000) To err is human: Building a safer health system. Institute of Medicine Washington, D.C.: National Academy Press.

Kraman, S. and Hamm, G. (1999). Risk management: Extreme honesty may be the best policy. Annals of Internal Medicine, 131(12

Liebman, C. B. & Hyman, C. (2004). A mediation skills model to manage disclosure of errors and adverse events to patients. Health Affairs 23

Lipsky, D et al; (1996) Emerging Systems for Managing Workplace Conflict: Lessons from American Corporations for Managers and Dispute Resolution Professionals. Jossey-Bass Publishers. Wiley Press NY

Love, L, Stulberg, J (2013) The Uses of Mediation from The Negotiator's Field book: The Desk reference for the Experienced Negotiator. Chapter 66

Lamb, R. et al. (2003) Reconceptualizing Users as Social Actors in Information Systems Research. MIS Quarterly Vol. 27(2)

Lang, M. & Taylor, A. (2000). The making of a mediator: Developing artistry in practice. Jossey-Bass Publishers; San Francisco, CA.

Lewicki, R. & Benedict Bunker, B. , (1995) in Conflict cooperation and justice: Essays inspired by the work of Morton Deutsch. Jossey Bass, Inc.; San Francisco, CA.

Malhotra, D and Bazerman, M (2007) Negotiation Genius: How to Overcome Obstacles and Achieve Brilliant Results at the Bargaining Table and Beyond. Harvard Business School. Random House Publishing

Massachusetts General Hospital (2006). When things go wrong: Responding to adverse events. A consensus statement of the Harvard Hospitals. Massachusetts Coalition for the Prevention of Medical Errors. US Department of Health and Human Services. PSNET https://psnet.ahrq.gov/resources/resource/3474/when-things-go-wrong-responding-to-adverse-events

Marshall, P, Robson, R (2005) Preventing and Managing Conflict: Vital Pieces in the Patient Safety Puzzle. Healthcare Quarterly Vol 8

Mayer, B (2000) The Dynamics of Conflict Resolution: A Practitioner's Guide. Jossey-Bass, San Francisco, CA.

Mayer, B. (2004) Beyond Neutrality Confronting the crisis in conflict resolution. Wiley Press. San Francisco, CA

Mayer, B. (2012). The Dynamics of Conflict: A Guide to Engagement and Intervention (2nd ed.) Wiley Press. San Francisco, CA

Maxfield, D et al: The Silent Treatment Why Safety Tools and Checklists Aren't Enough to Save Lives. Vital Smarts, AORN, & AACN. https://www.psqh.com/analysis/the-silent-treatment-why-safety-tools-and-checklists-arent-enough/

Mazor, K., Simon, S., Gurwitz, J. (2004). Communicating with patients about medical errors: A review of literature. Archives of Internal Medicine, 164

McFarlane, J (2011) Dispute Resolution. Readings and Case Studies. 3rd edition Emond Montgomery publications, Toronto Canada.

Mclaughlin, J. (1986) Enforcement of Arbitral Awards under the New York Convention-Practice in U.S. Courts. Berkeley Journal of International Law (3)

Mediate. Com http://mediate.com/

Mediators Beyond Borders.
http://www.mediatorsbeyondborders.org/index.shtml

Menkel-Meadow, C. (1985), Transformation of Disputes by Lawyers: What the Dispute Paradigm Does and Does Not Tell Us, Journal of Dispute Resolution 25

Mills, M: (2002) Conflict in Health Care Organizations, Journal of Health Care Law and Policy 502.

Mnookin, R et al, (2003) Strategic Barriers to Dispute Resolution: A Comparison of Bilateral and Multilateral Negotiations. Journal of Institutional and Theoretical Economics (159)

Monk, G., Sinclair, S., & Nelson, M. (2015). Healthcare Professionals' Use of Narrative Mediation to Address Disclosure and Apology in the Aftermath of Medical Errors. Conflict and Narrative: Explorations in Theory and Practice, (3)

National Round Table on Environment and Economy. (1993). Building consensus for a sustainable future. Ottawa, Canada.
http://www.mediate.com/articles/consen.cfm.

Owen, H. (1992). Open space technology: A user's guide. Abbott Publishing; Potomac, MD.

Patel, M. (2015) Reframe Shift the Way You Work, Innovate, and Think. Lioncrest Publishing

Peacemakers Trust: http://www.peacemakers.ca/

Pranis, K., Stuart, B., Wedge, M. (2003). Peacemaking circles: From crime to community. Living Justice Press; St. Paul, MN.

Prehn, Anette.(2014) The Neuroscience of Reframing.
https://www.udemy.com/the-neuroscience-of-reframing-and-how-to-do-it/learn/v4/overview

Ragone, A., et al. (2006). Propositional-logic approach to one-shot multi issue bilateral negotiation. ACM SIGecom Exchanges (5).

Riskin, L. and Welsh, N (2008) Is That All There Is? 'The Problem' in Court-Oriented Mediation . George Mason Law Review, Vol. 15
Roth, Hyman and Stillman. (11/2016) American Arbitration Associations Advanced Training in Healthcare Mediation conference. San Francisco CA.

Roth, M and Fromer. L (2013) Identifying and resolving disputes in new accountable care settings AHLA Connections Vol 17
Schein, E. (1988). Process consultation: Its role in organization development 2nd Ed. Addison Wesley; Reading, MA.

Quinn-Schmitt, K (2011) Important Conversations. Springs Mediation, kerri@springsmediation.com.

Schorr, A. The Web-Savvy Patient: An Insider's Guide to Navigating the Internet When Facing Medical Crisis . The Patient Empowerment Network. ISBN: 1456324993

Schuman, S. (1996) The role of facilitation in collaborative groups. In Creating collaborative advantage. Sage Publications; Thousand Oaks, CA.

Schwarz, R.M. (2002). The skilled facilitator: New and revised edition. Jossey-Bass Publishers; San Francisco, CA.

Schwarz, R., et al. (2005). The skilled facilitator fieldbook: Tips, tools, and tested methods for consultants, facilitators, managers, trainers, and coaches. Jossey-Bass Publishers; San Francisco, CA.

Sonnenwald, D.(1996). Communication roles that support collaboration during the design process. Design Studies, 17

Smith, M. K. (2005). Bruce W. Tuckman - forming, storming, norming and performing in groups, the encyclopedia of informal education at www.infed.org/thinkers/tuckman.htm.

Stahl, G. (2000). A Model of Collaborative Knowledge-Building. In B. Fishman & S. O'Connor-Divelbiss Fourth International Conference of the Learning Sciences. Mahwah, NJ.

Stone, D.et al (2010). Difficult Conversations: How to Discuss What Matters Most. Penguin Publishing Group. NY

Susskind, L. & Cruikshank, J. (2006) Breaking Robert's Rules: The new way to run your meeting, build consensus, and get results. Oxford University Press; New York, NY.
Susskind, L., McKearnan, S., Thomas-Larmer, J. (1999). The consensus building handbook: A comprehensive guide to reaching agreement. Sage Publishers. Thousand Oaks, CA.

Tannen, D. (2013). That's Not What I Meant! How Conversational Style Makes or Breaks Relationships (1st ed.) First Harper press, NY.

Tarrant, C.(2018) Continuity and Trust in Primary Care: A Qualitative Study Informed by Game Theory. Annals of Family Medicine

Tarrant C, Stokes T, Colman AM. (2004) Models of the medical consultation: opportunities and limitations of a game theory perspective. Qual Safe Health Care (13)

Thompson, J. (2012). The Wheel of Conflict. https://www.psychologytoday.com/blog/beyond-words/201204/the-wheel-conflict

Tuckman, B & Jensen, M (1977). Stages of Small-Group Development Revisited. Group & Organization Management, (2)

Ury, W, Fisher R. (1992). Getting past no: Negotiating with difficult people. William New Edition London. Century Business
United States Institute of Peace http://www.usip.org/index.html

Yang, D., et al (2008). A Wiki Based System for Collaborative Requirements Negotiation. Proceedings of the 41st Annual Hawaii International Conference on System Sciences.

Zimmerman, B., Lindberg, C. & Plsek, P. (2001). Edgeware: Insights from complexity science for health care leaders (2nd ed.). Irving, TX: VHA.

ABOUT THE AUTHOR

Dr. Michael Schneider MD, FACS, MS-ADR is a board-certified neurosurgeon with thousands of surgeries and several academic appointments in his 30-year medical career. He graduated cum laude in 1983 from the University of Southern California with a bachelor's major in Biological Sciences with emphasis in genetic engineering. Dr Schneider entered medical school and graduated as an Alpha Omega Alpha recipient from the Keck-USC School of medicine in 1987 and completed his residency and fellowship in neurological surgery by 1994. He has practiced medicine in three academic positions, private practice and for the Veterans Healthcare Administration during his medical career. Dr. Schneider's legal education includes a master's degree from Creighton University School of Law. Dr. Schneider has served as chief of surgery, chief of neurosurgery, medical staff president, utilization review counsel, and worked extensively as an impartial facilitator in dispute resolution with human resources in several healthcare institutions.

Dr. Schneider's experience with hospital boards and medical staff developed expertise in risk management analysis and mitigation and he currently practices as a successful co-mediator and subject matter expert co-arbitrator, critical to litigation management. His unique perspective assures the litigation team avoids costly mistakes during liability prosecution, medical board actions and he is adept at resolving insurmountable conflicts between competitive and adverse healthcare professionals. Dr Schneider is particularly skilled as a facilitator during medical malpractice litigation.

Dr Schneider is a fierce advocate for fair and objective representation and works extensively with healthcare providers to mitigate the "second victim" syndrome. In his facilitator and coaching practice, Dr Schneider recognizes the caustic impact of adverse actions against practitioners and is committed to the concept that no provider feels abandon during legal proceedings.

Dr Schneider is an avid expert downhill skier and advanced open water rescue scuba diver with over one thousand dives throughout the world. He is a former Eagle Scout , Chapter Chief for Order of the Arrow, and former instructor for the Boulder Outdoor Survival School in Southern Utah (BOSS). Dr Schneider served as a USAF Officer and neurosurgeon, honorably discharge in 1997.

Dr Schneider is married for over 26 years to a successful spouse who is an NICU nurse, a trained professional Chef, author, best friend and closest confidant. Dr Schneider's three adult children are his greatest accomplishment.

Future publications.

Dr Schneider is the author of two additional books in this series. These books are designed to augment the healthcare providers education and preparation for the non-medical events that threaten clinical practices and professional fulfillment.

Both will be published in 2018.

Titles:

The Healthcare Practitioner's Guide to Litigation Management

The Healthcare Practitioner's Guide to Administrative Challenges
Navigating peer review, medical staff inquiry, medical and specialty board complaints and contested case hearings.

Feel free to contact Dr Michael Schneider at:

Provider Resolutions, LLP
315 S Coast Hwy 101 Ste U-102
Encinitas, CA 92024

www.provider-resolutions.com
omnineuro@gmail.com
linkedin.com/in/michael-schneider-md-ms-adr

www.ingramcontent.com/pod-product-compliance
Lightning Source LLC
Chambersburg PA
CBHW061139220326
41599CB00025B/4289